Myths, Madness and the Family

Myths, Madness and the Family

The Impact of Mental Illness on Families

David W. Jones

Consultant Editor: Jo Campling

palgrave

First published 2002 by
PALGRAVE
Houndmills, Basingstoke, Hampshire RG21 6XS and
175 Fifth Avenue, New York, N.Y. 10010
Companies and representatives throughout the world

PALGRAVE is the new global academic imprint
of St. Martin's Press LLC Scholarly and Reference Division and
Palgrave Publishers Ltd (formerly Macmillan Press Ltd).

ISBN 0–333–77618–6 paperback

This book is printed on paper suitable for recycling and
made from fully managed and sustained forest sources.

A catalogue record for this book is available
from the British Library.

10   9   8   7   6   5   4   3   2   1
11 10 09 08 07 06 05 04 03 02

Printed and bound by J. W. Arrowsmith Ltd., Bristol

Contents

Contents

Acknowledgements

There are a number of people whose help has been invaluable in allowing this book to see the light of day.

I am firstly indebted to Dylan Tomlinson's friendship and creative diplomacy for making the original project possible. The research was supported by the late North East Thames Regional Health Authority and by a grant from the Economic and Social Research Council. Professor Shulamit Ramon provided invaluable support throughout the development of the project.

There are a number of people who have provided advice, support and encouragement at different times. Thanks to Nick Wright for a great deal of support in the earlier stages, and to Helen Hingley-Jones and Anne Chappell on the recent versions. I must thank Jo Campling for help and encouragement in getting this to publication.

My greatest debt is towards the people who talked to me, and told me about their experiences. I am sure that speaking as openly as they often did to a complete stranger was not without cost. I hope I can repay that effort by representing their stories and experiences as well as I can in the hope that families in similar situations in the future may be better understood.

Finally, I dedicate this book to Isobel and Ben.

Introduction

I.1 The Struggle for Meaning

Carol Peters was interviewed as part of the study that informs many of the later chapters of this book. She is in her mid thirties and is married with two small children. She is also the sister of Donald, a man who has been treated for many years by the psychiatric services, having been diagnosed as suffering from schizophrenia.

In the passage below, Carol expresses her frustration with professional mental health workers, followed by a series of poignant questions. The frustration and the subsequent questions can be regarded as an appeal for meaning.

There is anger at professionals for seeming to withhold meaning, by refusing to 'label the illness' (1). Contrast is made with 'normal nursing', and the apparent predictability of the course and treatment of cancer (2). Then there is the appeal for meaning, articulated through a series of questions (3), voiced in the face of the distress caused by the apparently irrational and deeply troubling behaviour (4).

But they [professionals] also have this idea that they don't label the illness [1], they don't like to label the illness so... they won't tell you what it is – that he's just ill. You see, it's probably something in their training that they've got... It should be taken as far back as when they're all being trained for these jobs, as to how to deal with the families. I mean in normal nursing [2], when you're dealing with... like my father-in-law when he had that brain tumour, the nurse was wonderful with us. She took us into a room, she explained exactly what was happening, the fact that it was malignant; what was going to happen to him – at 76 hours he would be this – but that during that time he wouldn't have any recollection. She went through the whole bit. Now that's what you need in mental illness... You need somebody who will sit down and you can say: 'How can we deal with this? How are we meant to react? What do you want us to do?' [3] We can only be there for Donald, and you go through these stages where Donald thinks he hasn't got a family, he doesn't want to know you, he'll throw you out of the place, he'll scream at you, he'll shout at you – you need

somebody. When times like that happen, you know you're not
immune to it all – it hurts [4]. 'We know he's ill. Can you explain to us
what is going on in his brain that he is suddenly screaming and shouting
at us, and abusing us and everything else, do you know why? ... What
can be done about it? And what do you want us to do about it?' –
except make nuisances of ourselves, with both them and with him,
because that's what you feel like.

This book is about the experiences of people like Carol who have a
relative who suffers from severe mental health problems. Such a book
cannot avoid being concerned with the relatives' distress, and the difficulties that they face. It is also about their struggle for meaning in the
face of what appears to be the breakdown of reason that we call madness. An important theme of the book is that their struggle is exacerbated by their finding that those experiences and their understanding of
those experiences cannot be shared with many people around them.
There is a degree of isolation experienced by families caused in part by
social attitudes that stigmatize mental illness, and in part by the attitude
of professionals who have often blamed families. Families have been
significant objects of psychiatric discourse, with aspects of family life
being seen as key to mental health and illness. Another important
theme of this book, however, is that families themselves are by no
means simply passive objects of psychiatric discourse, but are very active in defining sanity and madness. It is not only the families themselves
that will benefit if mental health professionals had a better understanding of their experiences. It will be argued through this book that the
attitudes and beliefs of the relatives are effectively helping to shape the
world in which mental illnesses are defined and understood. Through
understanding the perception of families we are reaching a better
understanding of the 'problem' of mental illness. Given the obvious
shifts in European and US mental health policies that have seen the
care of people with mental health problems being shifted from the
large mental hospitals towards the community, those families are likely
to have an increasingly large part to play.

I.2   The Policy Background

Across governments in Europe and America there are clear intentions
to transfer the care of people with long-term mental health problems to
more community-based settings (Carrier and Tomlinson 1996; Murphy

1991; Tomlinson 1992). In England and Wales the number of people living in the large mental hospitals, or 'asylums', has been in decline since the 1950s (Tooth and Brooke 1961). The 1990 NHS and Community Care Act (DoH 1990) made these intentions very explicit (Ramon 1985). Despite such apparently bold and forthright intentions, there has remained a great deal of public confusion surrounding the future direction of mental health policies within Community Care. In the early 1990s, Ramon (1992: xvi) was able to say:

> What is striking in the current public debate on mental health services in Britain, Italy and the USA is the relative lack of vigour in defending hospitals or calling for their reinstatement, coupled with considerable scepticism that care in the community can work for people with serious mental health problems.

A series of very public crises involving people suffering from long-term mental health problems (Muijen 1996) led to a series of controversial policy measures, such as Community Supervision and Supervision Registers, in the UK (DoH 1993, 1994; Eastman 1997; Parkin 1996; Vaughan 1998). The importation of the Care Programme Approach from the USA, which had been developed there partly in response to concerns about hospital closure, also served to highlight a degree of ambivalence (DoH 1994, 1995a–c).

There still seems to be an absence of clear alternatives being presented by critics. On the one hand there are voices complaining of 'community neglect' (Scull 1984), and calling for more psychiatric beds and for the closure programmes to be halted (witness the prominent campaigning by *Schizophrenia: A National Emergency* (SANE) described by Ramon 1991; see also Weller 1985). On the other hand, alarms have been raised about the threat posed to civil liberties by increasingly coercive powers being handed to psychiatrists and other mental health professionals (Baker 1997), or objections made to the re-creation of repressive psychiatric institutions in the community (Sullivan 1998).

The persistent ambiguity is particularly evident when the group of people who might be called the 'new long-stay' population are considered. These are the relatively young people whose lives might have been spent largely in the asylums, were they not closing. Their apparent plight has cast something of a shadow over the formerly optimistic reports of asylum closures in North America (Harding et al. 1987; Mosher and Burti 1989; Warner 1985) and Britain (TAPS 1989, 1990). Studies suggest that they have significant levels of social impairments and are prone to suffer multiple deprivations in terms of unemployment, homelessness (or inadequate housing), and social isolation (Babiker 1980; Bewley et al. 1981; Christie-Brown, Ebringer and Freedman 1977; Ebringer and Christie-Brown 1980; Freeman and Choudrey 1984; Holcomb and Ahr 1987; Mann and Cree 1976; Measey and Smith 1973; Pepper, Ryglewicz and Kirshner 1982; Rud and Noreik 1982; Schwartz and Goldfinger 1981; Todd, Bennie and Carlisle 1976). This is the group for whom the question about what is replacing the hospitals is most poignantly raised. Can they be *cared* for within the community (Carrier and Tomlinson 1996)?

I.3   The Caring Community?

A key distinction has been made at a policy level between informal and formal care (Bulmer 1987). Formal care is that which is provided, usually by professional workers, by the state or its institutions. Informal care is that which is thought to exist 'naturally' in the community. Informal care networks, ideally, consist of the extended family, friends and neighbours. The assumption is increasingly being made, supported by evidence, that families actually provide the vast bulk of informal care in cases of chronic illness or disability (Alcock 1996; Bulmer 1987; Cowen 1999). Feminist writers have noted the predominance of women carers (Finch and Groves 1984; Land 1978; Ungerson 1990; Wilson 1977). Whilst full recognition of the contribution made by informal carers has become more prominent, as witnessed by the implementation of the 1995 Carers' Act in the UK, for example (DoH 1995), there has still been remarkably little work that seeks to understand the complex and often psychological aspects of caring (Lloyd 2000). As will be argued in this book, there have been strong ideological reasons for the particular neglect of the families' perspective in the area of mental illness. It will be argued that an understanding of the families' experiences has been a neglected dimension not only of the policy debate, but also of the models that professionals bring to their work with families. We know little about the perceptions and experiences of the families of those younger people who need to develop lives outside of hospital if asylum closure is to be a success.

I.4   The Relationship between Family and Psychiatry

It will be argued that part of the difficulty that we have had in forging new policies for people with serious mental illnesses has been the failure to analyse adequately the relationship between families and psychiatry. The first two chapters of this book will explore some of the different ways that families have been significant targets of critical professional attention. Many psychiatric and psychological models have supposed that families are causing mental illness. What is interesting is the way that the many critics of psychiatry (Miller 1986) have failed to examine this assumption; it was indeed taken up with enthusiasm by R. D. Laing (Laing 1959; Laing and Esterson 1964), who was such an important figure in the British anti-psychiatry movement (Sedgwick 1982). It is partly in order to understand the complicated relationship that exists between psychiatry and 'the family' that the metaphor of the myth of the family is invoked.

I.5   The Myth of the Family

This book makes use of the metaphor of the family as a 'myth'. The argument is that myths about the power of families to do great harm – or to heal and make all things well – sweep through policy assumptions, the models used by professionals and academics, *and* through the lives of ordinary people. By myth, it is not meant that these ideas are simply untrue, but that many assumptions about the significance of 'family' have become so culturally embedded and 'obvious', or commonsensical, that they are not questioned (Barthes 1973; Lévi-Strauss 1968). The notion of 'family' is an important organizing feature in our perceptions, our identities and our culture. An important message of the book is that the contemporary family has to be understood in these terms. There has been a great deal of (sometimes heated and anguished) debate about the changing structure and functions of families (see McRae 1999 for a significant review of various aspects of the changing family in the UK). The increasing rates of divorce, separation and single-parenthood are sometimes put forward as representing the demise of the family (Poponoe 1993). The model of family relationships being put forward here would suggest that these criticisms are misplaced. The people interviewed, whose experiences form the core of this book, reflect the range and diversity of the urban North London population from which they came. Over half the sample were from ethnic minorities, mainly Afro-Caribbean (see King et al. 1994 for discussion of the over-representation of ethnic minorities in the psychiatric system). Some people interviewed were married and in conventional nuclear families. Some were divorced, some were single parents, widowed, separated or single. Yet they all seemed to have in common the idea that 'family' meant something extremely powerful to them. It seemed to mean something in ways that words could not always describe; in ways that could not be readily attributed, for example, to the rules of reciprocity and obligation that have become the currency of the very rationalistic models that have been in vogue to describe family and kin relations (Finch and Mason 1993). It is also notable that a great deal of effort in the social sciences has gone into studying 'the family' in terms of the relationships between parents and young children and relatively little into studying family relationships between adults (Bornat et al. 1999; Greene and Boxer 1986). Yet the experiences of these people suggest that family relationships between adults, in the absence of children, can be extremely important (Greenberg, Kim and Greenley 1997). Similar points have been raised by those studying 'new' family forms, such as gay or 'families of choice' (Weeks, Heaphy and Donovan 1999).

I.6   The Challenge of the Study of the Family and Mental Illness

Part of the original motivation for this book was to reach a greater understanding of the relationship of mental illness to family life. It will be argued that study of families presents a challenge not only because the family is a complex and multifaceted creature but also because there are ideals (or fantasies) about family life which run through research models, policy assumptions, professional models, and people's everyday expectations. These ideals make understanding of real, ordinary families a challenge. This book, therefore, has several related purposes:

- To examine the experiences of relatives of people who have come to be seen as suffering from severe mental illness in such a way that the meanings that events hold, and the emotional aspects of events and relationships, can be captured.

- To offer insight into the experiences of those families in order that those concerned with formulating and implementing mental health policies may be better able to work constructively with those families. This book, in many ways, is presenting the relatives' points of view. These views are sometimes diametrically opposed to those presented by people who have experience of mental illness and the psychiatric services (Lawson 1991; Reed and Reynolds 1996). There is no claim being made that the relatives' view is *the* correct way to view mental illness, but it is how events are understood by relatives. People who are engaging and working with families need to appreciate their point of view.

- To trace the influence of families and ideas about families in the mental health system. On the one hand, ideas about families have influenced the research models and policy aims, whilst on the other, families themselves have shaped practices through their own responses to mental illness.

I.7   Overview of the Book

Chapter 1 ('The Family, the Asylum and Community Care') charts the influence of ideas about families within the broad sweep of social and mental health policies that have nurtured and are now undermining the asylums. It will be argued that the significance of the assumed relationship between family and mental illness was evident in the reasoning for the growth of the asylums in the nineteenth century. Anxiety about the damage posed to individuals by failing families was one justification for the construction of asylums. It was also hoped that an idealized familial-style environment, in the shape of 'moral treatment' within the asylums, would prove therapeutic. It will also be argued that families were active participants in the asylum movement, since they used them to place relatives with whom they struggled to cope. Families were thus involved in the very identification of mental illness. This theme of families themselves being involved in the definition of sanity and madness is an important one that will be picked up in the later chapters that examine the experiences of contemporary families. What becomes clear from families themselves is how important familial ideals are in the definition of sanity. It can also be argued that families have played a part in the demise of the asylums through their ideological place in the welfare state and the policies of community care.

The assumption that family life is bound up with the distinction between sanity and insanity has led to a great volume of research on families and mental illness. The overview of this research provided in Chapter 2 ('Observing the Family') makes it clear that the principal research paradigms, like asylum and community care policies, have been shaped by quite ideologically informed assumptions and anxieties about family life. Little attempt has been made to understand the families' perspectives. This is despite the fact that there have been discernible moves toward the seeking of the views of 'ordinary participants' in social research for some decades now. As early as the 1950s, for example, Erving Goffman spent time in gaining an understanding of the inmates' and staff's view of the psychiatric asylum (Goffman 1961). Despite such moves, as Chapter 2 stresses, although there have been many studies of 'families and mental illness', they have generally been of a very different ethos. They have usually not been seeking to understand the families' experiences or communicate their point of view. Chapters 3 to 8 therefore address this gap in knowledge. These chapters have largely been informed by interviews carried out by the author. Given the book's reliance on material gathered from this research, the methodology is described in some detail at the end of Chapter 2.

Chapter 3 ('The Complicated Grief') illustrates an important common feature of the relatives' experiences. They all felt that the person who had become 'ill' had suffered a great change, as if they had become someone else, or their real self had been covered up. Therefore, the families were all dealing with a loss, which can be usefully understood in terms of a complex bereavement process.

Another feature of the relatives' experiences which (perhaps more surprisingly) was relatively uniform was the way in which people made recourse to forms of medical model in order to understand what had happened to their family member. An obvious explanation for this might be that the families had simply absorbed ideas from the psychiatric services with whom they were in contact. Chapter 4 ('The Relationship with Psychiatry and Psychiatric Knowledge') explores the families' views of psychiatry and medical services and casts doubt on this explanation. The families very often reported bad experiences with professionals. Tales of poor communication and of scepticism about psychiatric models and treatments were common.

Chapter 5 ('The Moral Construction of Diagnosis') goes on to explore the models of illness that people are using. It will be argued that the models used were influenced by some of the complex feelings and the webs of social relationships in which people were engaged. In constructing theories about causes of illness, there was often a deep concern with moral responsibility. It was also apparent that people's ideas about mental illness were being influenced by their own very powerful (yet often unacknowledged) feelings of anger, guilt and shame.

The importance and complexity of the emotion of shame and the experience of stigma will be explored further in Chapter 6 ('Coping with Stigma: The Significance of Shame and Identity'). The emotion of shame is one that has only recently been subject to much serious study.

It will be argued that consideration of the emotion of shame helps elucidate the experience of stigma. It will be suggested that stigma and shame must be understood as both social and psychological processes. Feelings of shame can be triggered by social disapproval, but they can also occur in the absence of overt social processes, being triggered by internal psychological events. A number of strategies that people had developed for coping with the threat posed by such alarming feelings will be investigated. It will be further argued that the ways in which these relatives seemed to experience threats to their identities by having a family member suffer from mental illness suggests something important about the significance of family relationships. The great commitment that some of these relatives showed for one another might be better explained in terms of the identifications they have with one another, rather than by reference to more abstract rules, such as 'obligation' or 'reciprocity', which have been used to explore kinship relations (Finch and Mason 1993).

The theme is developed further in Chapter 7 ('The Myth of the Family'), where it will be argued that the ideas about 'the family' function as a myth. By this is meant that it operates as an explanatory device, within the bounds of which certain premises are not questioned. The idea of the family provides apparently uncomplicated explanations for relationships that are often made up of highly irrational processes concerning aspects of human experience, such as sexuality and emotion, that have been most troubling for rational accounts. It is here that the roots of the entwined relationship between ideas of sanity, madness and family are located.

Chapter 8 ('Managing Myths: Reaching New Understandings') examines the ways that people have of coping with the complex feelings they have and with the standards imposed by ideals of family life. It will be argued that it may be possible to characterize a process whereby people can come to certain levels of acceptance and accommodation. In reaching situations of reasonable equilibrium powerful feelings of ambivalence have to be reconciled. What emerges as important is that new understandings seem to emerge from processes of dialogue and negotiation. This negotiation needs to take place between relatives, professionals and, crucially, with the 'identified patient' themselves.

Ultimately this book aims to be a contribution to the dialogue we need to have about serious mental illness if new and better understandings and solutions are to emerge. It is in no way a balanced account. For example, the views of the users of mental health services do not appear here at all. This is quite simply because their voices are beginning to be heard through the medium of research (Barham and Hayward 1991; Rogers, Pilgrim and Lacey 1993) and in their own right (Lawson 1991; Reed and Reynolds 1996). This book attempts to be a step towards getting the voices of relatives heard in the discussion. Quite extensive quotes from the families are used throughout, partly in order to give these families a voice, but also to give those who might find themselves working with similar families an idea of the quite subtle and sometimes rather covert ways that many issues might emerge.

1

The Family, the Asylum and Community Care

This chapter will spell out why consideration of the world of the 'family' is so important to our understanding of serious mental illness. It will be argued that families, for various reasons, have been a significant factor in the lives of those who have come to be seen as suffering from serious mental illness. It is not only the actual behaviour of families but, perhaps even more importantly, it is also the ideas and assumptions about 'the family' that have been such critical features of the environment which has shaped not just the policies and practices that are aimed at mental illness, but our very definitions of sanity and madness.

Little consideration has been given to the role that families have played in the history of psychiatry. This is despite a large and contentious literature on the differing explanations for the development of modern psychiatry, which was most visibly represented by the growth of the asylums during the eighteenth and nineteenth centuries (Alldridge 1979; Arieno 1989; Castel 1988; Chesler 1972; Doerner 1981; Foucault 1967; Grob 1983, Hunter and Macalpine 1963; Jones 1972; Porter 1987; Rothman 1971; Scull 1979; Skultans 1979; Tomes 1994; Walton 1985). Two alternative accounts of the rapid development of the asylums may be characterized. The first holds that the asylums were conceived as places where people could be cared for and treated (Hunter and Macalpine 1963; Jones 1972). They were built in response to the belief that the varieties of insanity were potentially understandable and treatable diseases. The second, critical, account sees the asylums as emerging from increasingly sophisticated systems of classifying and controlling various forms of deviance (Ingleby 1985). According to this story, the asylums were part of the same system as the workhouse and prison; they were places where those whose behaviour threatened the social order could be gathered together and controlled (Foucault 1967; Scull 1979).

No attempt will be made to review this literature on the birth of psychiatry. There is no doubt that there are a number of complex social and historical reasons for the development of psychiatry and the asylums. The point will be made here, however, that the role of 'families' and familial ideologies are notable factors that have been largely neglected. The case being made here is in keeping with views that suggest that in order to fully understand the development of our responses to mental illness we need to look beyond the most visible aspects of official policy (in this case the asylums themselves) towards the wider social processes involved in shaping our constructs of insanity (Bartlett and Wright 1999).

In this chapter, it will be argued that ideological assumptions about the significance of family life have informed the models that have been used to understand and treat mental illness. This will help explain the paradox, explored further in Chapter 2, that a great volume of research has been carried out on 'families and mental illness', but very little of it gives us insight into what it is like for those families. Much of the research has been driven by quite specific ideological concerns (such as anxiety about gender roles in families). At the same time it must be appreciated that families are not merely passive objects being pushed around by ideological forces or professional interests. Families themselves have been active in shaping responses towards mental illness. Historical evidence suggests that they did this in a very tangible way by deciding to use the asylums to place their relatives who they deemed to be insane. One historian has thus described the families as the 'patrons of the asylums' (Tomes 1994). This historical perspective is important in that it alerts us to be aware that the actions of families may well be a factor that shapes the alternatives to those asylums. Indeed, this is an important theme of the later chapters that are concerned with the experiences of contemporary families. Families can be very active in engaging with and appropriating ideas about mental illness.

1.1   Family Ideology and Madness

Some historical perspective is required for understanding why the relationships between ideas of mental illness and family life are so entwined. Ideas about psychiatry and family life have, over the last few centuries in the West, evolved together because they are both institutions in which it is hoped people's emotional lives might be contained and controlled. This link emerged as people's emotional lives began to be regarded with increasing ambivalence. On the one hand, emotions were viewed as a significant aspect of the social order, providing the social glue between individuals and social institutions (Doerner 1981). Positive feelings of love and commitment were seen as providing social cohesion as the traditional order provided by feudal ties, religious authority and neighbourhood links fell away (Foucault 1979; Gillis 1985, 1987; MacDonald 1981; Rothman 1971). Also, feelings of ambition and endeavour came to be seen as important motors of industrial progress (Doerner 1981). On the other hand, there was still ambivalence towards powerful emotions as it was felt that they could threaten the social order if they were directed into rebellion and protest against the norms and authorities of the day. It was at this point of ambivalence that a link was forged between ideas of family and of mental illness. By the birth of the asylum era madness itself was coming to be seen as a failure of emotional control (Scull 1979; Skultans 1979). Both the family (Aries 1962; Foucault 1979) and psychiatry (Doerner 1981) were seen as actors who could play a role in the promotion and containment of emotion. The role that families played in providing ideals of conduct is a clear thread linking a number of influential models of mental illness through the nineteenth and twentieth centuries. During the nineteenth century the idea of the 'moral treatment' of mental illness, which incorporated the assumption that an orderly familial environment could help return people to sanity, was an important factor that was used to justify the development of a widespread network of asylums. During the twentieth century, the view that families were responsible for fostering sane conduct became explicit as 'dysfunctional' families were directly blamed for causing mental illness by a number of psychological models – notably the family therapy model (which will be discussed in Chapter 2).

1.1.1 Anxiety about the Amoral Family: Moral Treatment

By the end of the eighteenth century the family was widely perceived to be a crucial component of the newly emerging social order in Western Europe (Donzelot 1979; Foucault 1967; Seccombe 1992). Family life was seen as an institution that could instil discipline into growing children and could enforce responsible behaviour onto the parents. By the middle of the nineteenth century doubts about the ability of many families to fulfil these duties were rife. There was vigorous debate in England about the effects of industrialization and urbanization on the moral climate and upon family life in particular (Lewis 1984; Weeks 1981). Fears that overcrowded and anonymous urban life encouraged sexual relationships outside of marriage were prominent (Fletcher 1847: 193). Anxiety about 'inbreeding' amongst the poor was being linked to ideas of physical and mental degeneration (Castel 1988, for example, describes Morel's theory of degeneration and insanity – see also Pick 1989). Worry about gender roles became particularly discernible (Seccombe 1992; Weeks 1981) as the availability of factory work drew women out of the home to earn possibly more than men. This threatened to violate, according to Gaskell (1836: 89), 'all the decencies and moral observances of domestic life' (see also Jenkins 1874).

David Rothman's (1971) portrayal of the rise of the North American asylums lays great stress on the importance of this perception of the family as the crucial socializing force. He argues that this key duty fell upon the family during the early nineteenth century as communities were perceived to be more fragmented and the influence of the church declined. Reasoning then followed that if the family background of an individual was defective, that individual would fall into sin, crime and madness. If people had become insane (or criminal), the answer was to remove them from their defective families and sin-ridden communities and place them in institutions that could provide a setting in which people could learn a self-regulating discipline. Similar points emerge from Skultans's (1979) work on the importance given to the 'moral management' of the insane within English asylums.

The idea of the 'moral treatment' of madness was an important impetus to the growth of the asylums, as even Andrew Scull (1979), who is scathing about the ultimate form that the asylums took, acknowledges. The expectation of moral treatment was that if people were placed in an orderly environment and exposed to familial discipline they would be more likely to effect a recovery and would thus be able to return to a normal life. Samuel Tuke, one of the reformers credited with popularizing moral treatment, planned the York Retreat in England to provide a family-style environment, away from the corruption of the outside world. The residents were to be treated like children, subject to prompt punishments and rewards, taught that their behaviour had moral repercussions in that it disrupted the rest of 'the family' (Digby 1985; Doerner 1981; Skultans 1979). Daniel Tuke, writing in 1882, finished off a summation of the important aspects of the York Retreat by noting 'that from which the first has been regarded as a most important feature of the institution, is its homishness – the desire to make it a family as much as under the peculiar circumstances of the case is possible' (quoted in Skultans 1975: 154–5). Donnelly (1983: 46) argues that, although the Tukes were unusual in so directly associating the idea of 'family' with the asylum, 'moral pressures, exerted with a force close to the intensity of a parent's bond to a child, were the fundamental motor of the new plan of "management" in asylums and its most telling symptom'. The creation of dedicated, state-monitored asylums would allow for moral treatment to accomplish cure (after the fashion of the York Retreat and similar private establishments).

Therefore, it can be argued that anxiety about the moral state of the family helped promote and shape the growth of the asylum, and the emphasis on 'moral treatment'. Unfortunately, Scull (1979) and Rothman (1971) are able to report how quickly the reforming institutions, in England and North America respectively, degenerated into merely custodial ones. Chesler also highlights the importance given to 'family life' in the asylum. In her radical feminist story, however, there is no hint of any contradiction between 'moral treatment' and subjugation: 'mental asylums are families bureaucratised: the degradation and disenfranchisement of self, experienced by the biologically owned child (patient, woman) takes place in the anonymous and therefore guiltless embrace of strange fathers and mothers' (1972: 34).

1.1.2   Twentieth-Century Welfarism and Family Therapy

If anxiety about the family, and the implied power of family life, was influencing thought about mental illness during the era of asylum building, the influence on twentieth-century models of mental illness and practices is even clearer. The assumption that mental illnesses are caused by family life became very evident in the models of illness operating in psychiatry and psychology. Also, more general anxiety about the perils that might be faced if families were allowed to degenerate was manifest in the way the principles of welfarism aimed to buttress family life.

The population of the asylums in Britain reached a peak in 1954 and fell rapidly thereafter (Tooth and Brooke 1961). The demise has been subject to similar debate and controversy as the rise of the asylums. There is not the space to consider these theories, which range from considering the impact of innovations in medication (Clare 1976), or of new philosophies of care (Ramon 1985), to the view that governments began to find institutional care too costly (Scull 1984). Whilst there is no doubt merit in all these views, it will be argued here that it is important to understand that the demise of the asylums took place within the context of the development of the welfare state, which provided alternatives to institutional care for people with illnesses and disabilities. Within the welfare state there is a powerful commitment to the ideological significance of the family as the core unit of society. Certainly, the fall of the asylum population fits well chronologically with the establishment of the welfare state, which developed rapidly in Britain in the post-war years (Gough 1979). Some of the actions of the welfare state, such as the provision and subsequent targeting of public housing on poorer and marginalized groups (Malpass and Murie 1987), has helped the asylums to close by providing material support for people outside of the asylums.

1.1.3   Post-war Anxiety: the Family and the Welfare State

A highly significant impetus to the growth of the welfare state was the felt need to bolster the nuclear family (Deakin 1987; Hill 1993; Lewis 1992; Midwinter 1994; Wolfram 1987). Many family conflicts were being created as families were reunited after the Second World War (Turner and Rennell 1995), with the divorce rate in Britain and the USA reaching unprecedented levels that were only achieved again in the 1970s (Phillips 1988; Wolfram 1987). There was anxiety about the number of women in the workplace on both sides of the Atlantic, just as there had been in Britain a century before. In an effort to bolster traditional family forms, women were being encouraged out of the factories and back into the home (Lewis 1992).

These anxieties were part of a conducive environment that allowed a sufficient political consensus to nurture the growth of the welfare state (Gough 1979). Wilson (1977) argues that this growth had at its heart the reinforcement of 'traditional' gendered family relationships. Wilson (1977) and other feminist critics (Land 1978, for example) point out that many of the state's welfare activities are designed to buttress and support the family:

> First and foremost today the Welfare State means the State controlling the way in which the woman does her job in the home of servicing the worker and bringing up her children.   (Wilson 1977: 39)

The practical significance of the welfare state for people with disabilities, including serious mental illness, is that it provided social insurance and housing for non-working members of the community (Rose 1986). As disillusion with the ability of institutions to provide anything like family care set in (Barton 1959), so there was a shift towards seeing therapeutic value within the community itself (Bulmer 1987). Community care policy, seen as an evolution of state welfare strategies, puts very clear emphasis on the role of the family (Bulmer 1987; Busfield 1986; Finch and Groves 1984; Land 1978). The decline of the asylums has taken place on both sides of the Atlantic, therefore, in a period where government policies have been attempting to resource and strengthen the family in order that they can care for their 'own' dependants.

The sometimes quite subtle ideological importance given to the family within the specific workings of community care policy were picked up by Christine Perring (McCourt-Perring 1993; Perring 1990) in her study of the community care homes to which patients who had lived for many years in a large psychiatric hospital were moved. She noted that '[t]he model is one of a substitute family where carers are viewed in a quasi-maternal role, their managers as paternal and the residents as child-like' (Perring 1992: 161). Such observations emphasize the continuity between the ideals of nineteenth-century moral treatment and community care policies of the late twentieth century. The linkage being made between idealizations of family life and the promotion of 'mental health' is very clear.

1.1.4 Searching for the Cause of Mental Illness within the Family

Whilst the nineteenth-century principle of asylum-based 'moral treatment' is partly premised on the assumption that family life was somehow linked to madness, this became a transparent presumption by the middle of the twentieth century. In the period following the Second World War the spotlight of critical professional attention became conspicuously fixed on the family (Rose 1989). Family genes have been implicated, their behaviour assessed and their communication styles analysed by those who have assumed that the origins of mental illness lie somewhere within the family background of the sufferer (Biegel, Sales and Shulz 1990). The findings of those studies that have looked at families and mental illness will be considered in more detail in Chapter 2. The important point to be grasped here is that the research has been guided by highly ideological concerns that have led to considerable gaps in our understanding of the real experiences of families.

Theories that have placed the origins of mental illness within families have deep historical roots. Morel's nineteenth-century theory that insanity was the product of degenerate reproduction (that is, children produced by those with mental infirmity would be prone to mental illness) is a good example (Castel 1988). This idea has been taken up in a more sophisticated way by modern genetic models of transmission (McKenna 1997; Tsuang and Vandermey 1980) which place the origins of mental illness firmly within the family. More striking, though, was

the shift during the twentieth century towards a much more psychological perspective on the family (Rose 1989). The belief that family life
was constructed within the subjective worlds of feelings became obvious
in the tactics of those who believed that family life could be influenced
and improved through professional intervention (Dingwall, Eekelaar
and Murray 1983; Donzelot 1979; Parton 1991; Rose 1989; Stenson
1993; Timms 1964). Families became central for those constructing the
major psychological models of mental illness. Freud and psychoanalytic
theory are customarily seen as having established the principle of the
primacy of childhood experience as a determinant of psychological
health. Indeed, it was a psychoanalyst, Frieda Fromm-Reichman, who
coined the phrase 'schizophrenogenic mother' (Fromm-Reichman
1948). This is a mother who was seen as causing schizophrenia later in
her child's life by being emotionally very cold and withholding affection
from the child when a young baby. The vast majority of the psychoanalytic effort, however, has been applied to neurotic, rather than
psychotic, disorders. The fuller theorization of the familial causation of
psychosis took place mainly within the family therapy movement, which
has been responsible for the vast majority of the research on families
and mental illness.

1.1.5   Family Therapy and the Dysfunctioning Family

A group of researchers emerged in the post-Second World War period
who, although based in different research centres in the United States,
can collectively be called the early family therapists (see reviews by, for
example, Barker 1986; Nicholls and Schwartz 1991). They had the
common goal of hunting for the roots of schizophrenia in the behaviour
and communication styles of the immediate family (usually the parents)
of the identified patient. Here the linkage between ideals of family
behaviour and sanity become entirely explicit. The models they used
will be discussed in more detail in Chapter 2.

  The continuity with the preoccupations of the nineteenth-century
advocates of 'moral treatment' is striking. Sanity is seen as being nurtured
by the orderly conduct and clear communications occurring within the
family. That these ideas influenced the early work of the British anti-
psychiatry guru R. D. Laing (Laing 1959/1965; Laing and Esterson
1964) says a great deal about the comprehensiveness of the assumption.
Although Laing's own work had a radical edge of social criticism, the
exploration of the links between family and sanity undertaken by most
of the early family therapy researchers can be seen as being provoked

by familiar anxiety about the place of the family within the arena of social change – this time made clear by the upheaval of the Second World War in Europe and the United States.

Nathan Ackerman (one of the leading figures in early family therapy research), who was concerned to understand schizophrenia within the context of disordered family relationships, writing in 1958 had clear concerns about the direction and impact of social change:

> Blatantly in evidence are the disorganising trends in contemporary family life, the conflicts and failures of complementarity in man–wife relations, the signs of disintegration of the moral and ethical core of family relationships.   (Ackerman 1958: 335)

Here, plainly, we find anxiety about the disintegration of the family. As the above quotation would suggest, early family therapy case-studies often adhere to highly normative values of family functioning. Many ideological assumptions are made about gender roles in particular (see examples from Lidz and Bowen, in Chapter 2) which are often very explicit. Transgressions of traditional gender roles are seen as potential causes of poor mental health. Theodore Lidz, another important pioneer in family therapy research, was also motivated by anxiety about changing gender relations:

> It becomes increasingly evident scientifically, as it has been through common sense, that children require two parents with whom they interact and who optimally are of opposite sexes in temperament and outlook.... It appears that women having won their emancipation, recognise that women's self-realisation is linked to marriage and child bearing.   (Lidz 1963: 26)

The early family therapy literature has, not surprisingly, been criticized for its normative class, gender and ethnocentric values (Dell 1989; Perelberg and Miller 1990). The model is the two-parent nuclear family, with clear gender roles, any transgression from this being aberrant.

1.1.6   Active Families

So far the argument has been that, historically, families have been victims of ideological forces that have sought causes of insanity within the family. The case will now be made that families have not been merely passive objects of psychiatric discourse and theories. Families have also been quite active players in encouraging ideas about mental illness. This is particularly important to understand, as it will be argued through the rest of this book that contemporary families are key active participants in the world that shapes our understanding of mental illness.

Families were active partners in the asylum-building project, as they encouraged the proliferation of the asylums by using them to place their relatives. It was very often families that were deciding who was insane, who should be treated in asylums. Thus, through their activities many families played a part in the definition of madness during the asylum era.

The involvement of families in the confinement of their relatives in asylums has been directly studied by Walton (1985), MacKenzie (1992) and Suzuki (1999) in Britain, and Tomes (1994) in America. Walton examined records from the Lancaster County Asylum and argued that those admitted were 'not so much "inconvenient people" ... as impossible people in the eyes of families, neighbours, and authorities'. The asylum provided 'relief for desperate families rather than an easy option for the uncaring' (Walton 1985: 143). Nancy Tomes (1994) studied the development of the Pennsylvania Hospital for the Insane through the eighteenth and nineteenth centuries. As a result of analysis of letters written by relatives to the hospital staff, she argues that families were active partners in shaping the development of the asylum. Tomes refers to families as 'the patrons' of the asylums, since it was they who wanted somewhere to put their relatives with whom they were struggling to cope. Charlotte MacKenzie's (1992) study of the development of the private Ticehurst Asylum in England documents in detail the intimate involvement of family members in the decision to admit to the asylum, in the monitoring of treatment and the decision to discharge. She comments in her conclusion:

> Given the central role of the family in choosing forms of care, it is surprising that, with the exception of Tomes's study of Pennsylvania Hospital for the Insane, it is a dimension which has been relatively neglected in the histories of the asylum movement.
>
> (MacKenzie 1992: 214)

Whilst MacKenzie is surely right to draw attention to this neglect, there have been other studies that have observed families' involvement. Castel (1988) detailed the rights of families to have relatives detained in pre- and post-revolutionary France. Grob (1983: 9), in noting that most commitments to American asylums were by the families, observed: 'The diagnosis of insanity often did not involve the community. Nor were most commitments begun by law enforcement personnel. Proceedings were usually initiated by the immediate family.' The involvement of families in commitments to asylums has been noted in historical work on the New England Maclean Asylum (Jimenez 1987), and on confinements to the North Wales Lunatic Asylum during the nineteenth century (Hirst and Michael 1999). Work utilizing English asylum records (Arieno 1989) and Irish asylum records (Finnane 1996; Prior 1996) has also pointed to the active participation of families.

These historical observations are important. If families were actively involved in the creation of the asylums, we have to ask what role might they play in shaping the alternatives to those asylums?

1.2 Summary

Historical evidence has been put forward in this chapter to suggest that familial ideologies were an important spur to the development of the asylum movement. There was anxiety about the impact of social change on family life and gender roles in particular. The innovation of 'moral treatment', premised on the belief in the therapeutic benefit of familial-style discipline, was an important justification of the move to build asylums.

The demise of the asylums was encouraged by the provisions of the welfare state, which were aimed towards the bolstering of an idealized nuclear family. Subsequent moves to close the asylums have taken place within the context of community care policies which assume the positive involvement of families in the provision of care. Yet the latter part of the twentieth century is also a period that saw 'the family' come under scrutiny as a cause of mental illness. Much of our understanding of the relationship between families and mental illness has been shaped by these ideological concerns.

At the same time as being objects of these professional and policy interests, families themselves were actively engaging with the construction of practices directed towards mental illness. They were actively encouraging the proliferation of the asylums by using them to place their relatives who they felt were 'mentally ill'.

All this suggests that if we are to reach a better understanding of the contemporary world of serious mental illness, attention needs to be turned towards the families themselves. Certainly, if professionals are to consult and work in partnership with carers, as is often presumed even in legislation such as the 1995 Carers Act in Britain (DoH 1995), then they need to have a good understanding of their perspective. Yet, as Chapter 2 will emphasize, most of the research on families and mental illness has been driven by policy and ideological concerns rather than a wish to understand the perspective of those families (Hatfield and Lefley 1987).

2

Observing the Family

Reviews of the literature concerned with families and serious mental illness (Biegel, Sales and Shulz 1990; Hatfield and Lefley 1987; Perring, Twigg and Atkin 1990) reveal a great volume of research, but very little of it sheds light on the experience, or the perspective, of families (Cook, Pickett and Cohler 1997). This stands in contrast to the growing literature that explores the perspective of the mental health service user (Barham and Hayward 1991; Goldie 1986; Reed and Reynolds 1996; Rogers, Pilgrim and Lacey 1993; McCourt-Perring 1993). This deficiency can be understood by reference to the issues discussed in Chapter 1. Families tend to be viewed through highly ideological lenses, as they are assumed to have power to shape the subjective and affective lives of individuals (Donzelot 1980; Foucault 1979; Rose 1989) and they play such vital social roles (Lewis 1992; Wilson 1977). Too much of the research has been guided by those concerns, such that families have usually only been studied as objects of professionals' and policy makers' interests. This chapter will briefly outline the main areas of research on families and mental illness and will then describe the approach that guided the research that informs the subsequent chapters of the book.

The first part of this chapter will provide an overview of four areas of research on families and mental illness. The first of these is 'family therapy research', which is by far the largest body of work. The strong feature of this work is that it has sought the causes of serious mental illness in the behaviour and characteristics of the sufferers' families (Kreisman and Joy 1974). The second paradigm consists of the various 'psychoeducational approaches', which are forms of research that do not necessarily assume that families have caused the illness, but do suppose that family behaviour will impact on the course of the illness. The third research model supposes that families living with someone who suffers from mental illness carry 'a burden'. Various attempts have been made to measure that burden. The fourth section will review the relatively small number of studies that have taken a more explorative approach to understanding families' predicaments. The second part of the chapter describes the methodological approach taken by the study that informs the rest of the book.

2.1   Previous Research: the Family as an Object of Study

2.1.1   Family Therapy Research

This is the largest body of literature concerned with the families of people suffering from mental illness. In discussing family therapy here reference is not being made to all therapeutic efforts which might happen to be made with a family, but a quite specific construction of the family as being the cause of illness within one of its members (Barker 1986; Foley 1974; Kreisman and Joy 1974). Within this influential paradigm much effort has been expended in tracing the roots of schizophrenia within the families' behaviour.

Family therapy research began in America in the late 1940s and came to prominence through the 1950s and 1960s. The primary assumption of the early family therapy research was that schizophrenia, as a disease or a set of symptoms, was in some way being created within the environment of the family, particularly through the parental behaviour (Hatfield and Lefley 1987; Kreisman and Joy 1974). Much of the early research involved very intensive, acute observation of families where one member of the family, invariably one of the children (as an adolescent or young adult), had been diagnosed as suffering from schizophrenia. It will not be possible to review comprehensively the various schools of family therapy here. The history of the movement can be read in several accounts (Barker 1986; Foley 1974; Goldenburg and Goldenburg 1991; Hoffman 1981; Nicholls and Schwartz 1991).

Whilst there was not one inventor of the family therapy approach, certain names appear ubiquitous in the many histories of family therapy. There were the psychoanalytically trained psychiatrists, Theodor Lidz and Nathan Ackerman. The research team based at Palo Alto, originally led by Gregory Bateson and including Jay Haley, John Weakland and eventually Don Jackson, was also influential. Lyman Wynne and Murray Bowen came somewhat later, but developed concepts that have been influential. The various ideas underlying family therapy models can be considered under three, overlapping, categories: functionalism, emotional disturbance, and communication dysfunction.

(a) *Functionalism*

Functionalism underlies most schools of family therapy. This is consistent with the dominant paradigm of American sociology through the 1950s and after (Parsons and Bales 1955). The basic tenet of this functionalism was to view social groups as systems, with the various components of the system being understood by considering the roles that they fulfil in maintaining that system. In families with a member suffering mental illness, the family itself is considered as such a system. It is then assumed that the symptoms of the identified patient serve some purpose useful to the family system.

Functionalist thinking in family therapy theory can be illustrated by a typical example from Murray Bowen (1960). Bowen worked by looking in detail at the dynamics of the family relationships before him and then by attempting to alter them. In this account of family therapy, the identified patient is the young daughter, suffering from a psychotic breakdown. Bowen construed the 'real' problem as being the dysfunctional relationship between the parents, and not the daughter's psychosis. The mother and daughter were seen as being unhealthily involved with each other, with the daughter's 'illness' serving to draw attention away from the dysfunctional relationship between the parents (where the real problem was thought to lie). The values and gender norms which are operating here are instructive. The mother is described initially as 'over-adequate' (1); it is assumed that a healthier arrangement is that the father is head of the family (2). The mother is thought to emerge from the therapeutic process as a 'kind, motherly' figure (3):

> The father remained on the periphery in an inadequate position. Gradually the father began to participate in the family problems. The conflict shifted to the mother–father relationship. As the father began to take some stands against the over-adequate mother [1], she became much more anxious, challenging and aggressive towards him. Eventually he assumed a position as head of the family [2], in spite of her marked anxiety, tremulousness and protest. In a few days she rather quickly changed to a kind, motherly, [3] objective person. She said, 'It is so nice finally to have a man for a husband. If he can keep on being a man, then I can be a woman.' (Bowen 1960: 369)

Eventually, the parents became much closer, the daughter losing the 'close symbiotic relationship' with the mother and going on, according to Bowen (1960: 369) to 'make some solid progress'. This notion of the symptom serving a family system function has been taken up as a central principle of the later Milan systemic school (Boscolo et al. 1987).

(b) *Emotional disturbance*

Some of the leading protagonists in the family therapy movement (such as Bowen, Lidz and Jackson) were trained in psychoanalysis (Hoffman 1981). It is therefore not surprising to find that early family experiences were considered particularly significant in providing the foundations of mental health and illness. According to this perspective, schizophrenia was a response to emotional deprivation, such as the loss or absence of one or other parent, or the plain odd, eccentric behaviour of the parents.

A study by Lidz and Lidz (1949) provides a good example of this sort of study. They examined the family background of a number of schizophrenia patients and considered five different categories of factors which might be relevant: the loss of one parent through death or divorce; the incompatibility of parents (special emphasis seems to be given to religious differences); the instability of parents; particulars of parenting; and occurrences of mental illness in the family. Factors picked out for this particular group as possibly being relevant include everything from overt mental illness in the parents to such comments as:

> Father hypochondriacal and mother always nervous and irritable. Mother moody, thoughtless, rigid.

> Peculiar marriage of poor Protestant barber to wealthy Catholic heiress who was disowned and disinherited.

> Parents married only because of the pregnancy. No mutual life. Father took no interest in pat[ient] and found interests out of home. Mother silly.

Lidz and Lidz (1949: 343) concluded that 'study of the histories of these patients impresses forcefully that one patient after another was subjected to a piling up of adverse intrafamilial forces that were a major factor in moulding the misshapen personality...'. Through the focus on early family trauma the influence of psychoanalysis is clear.

(c) *Communication dysfunction*

Another way of looking at the families was as though they suffered from communication dysfunctions. According to this model schizophrenic symptoms were an inevitable result of confusing communications within the family. Gregory Bateson's theory of the 'double bind' is the best known example (Bateson et al. 1955). An archetypal scenario is the mother who asks her son why he does not show her affection, and when he goes to put his arm around her, she shrinks away from him. The son thus receives contradictory messages on different 'channels'. The overt verbal communication is 'come close to me', the covert (non-verbal) communication is 'stay away'. To Bateson and colleagues, a response to such confusion was for the son to develop the illogical thought processes characteristic of schizophrenia.

Summary of family therapy assumptions

The underlying idea shared by family therapy models was that family behaviour, usually parental behaviour, was causing the identified patient to suffer from schizophrenia. The family became an object under the gaze of the family therapists. There was no attempt to understand their perspectives (Reimers and Treacher 1995). Psychoanalytic ideas put the emphasis on early experience and family dynamics. The influence of cybernetic theory and functionalism allowed the relationships within the family to be analysed in terms of the parts they played in the functioning of the family system. Some of the mid-twentieth-century anxiety about gender roles, discussed in Chapter 1, are also apparent in the examples given above. The most damning criticism of the model is that the underlying belief that family behaviour caused schizophrenia went unquestioned in spite of the contrary evidence (Hirsch and Leff 1975). It is difficult to estimate the impact that the prevalence of these models had on relationships between families and professionals (Hatfield and Lefley 1987), but their presence might well help to explain the common findings of poor relationships between families and professionals that are discussed later (see also Howe 1989; Mashal, Feldman and Sigal 1989; Reimers and Treacher 1995).

Subsequent family therapy models have been less concerned with serious mental illnesses, such as schizophrenia. Those that have been interested in schizophrenia, such as the Milan school of systemic family therapy (Boscolo et al. 1987; Selvini-Palazzoli et al. 1978), and, of course, R. D. Laing (Laing 1959/1965; Laing and Esterson 1964) in Britain, have also carried these assumptions with them (see also Scott 1973; Scott and Ashworth 1967).

2.1.2   Psychoeducational Approaches

The psychoeducational approaches involve the provision of information, which is usually quite medically orientated, aimed to reassure the families that they are not to blame. These approaches do not involve research into the experience of families as such, although the fact that they take a more neutral stance is notable. Reviews of the success of the approaches paint a mixed picture, with Kazarian and Vanderheyden (1992) being rather equivocal about their efficacy, whilst Dixon and Lehman (1995) and Tarrier (1996) are more optimistic about their effectiveness.

(a)   *Expressed emotion*

The 'expressed emotion' (EE) approach can be regarded as the most research-led variant of the psychoeducational approaches. It has achieved a high profile, with many studies carried out and reported regularly in the psychiatric journals (Dixon and Lehman 1995; Leff 1994). Leff and Vaughan (1985) describe its development from an observation that people discharged from hospital with diagnoses of schizophrenia who returned to families were more likely to be readmitted than those discharged to other environments (Brown et al. 1966). They decided that the problem within some families was the expression of negative emotion and criticism and a high degree of emotional involvement (high expressed emotion: high EE). Having developed interview schedules to detect and measure the degree of EE, they found that where high EE was present the identified patient was more likely to relapse. Further work, which involved intervening and providing the family with advice about the illness and how to cope, suggested that where EE was decreased, the relapse rate was reduced (Leff 1994).

The EE researchers have been a lot more circumspect than family therapists about actually blaming the family for causing mental illness. They have still been criticized, however, for providing yet another stick with which to beat families. Hatfield (1987b: 61) argues that '[h]igh EE and low EE are seen as labels that once again depict families as "good families" and "bad families" – usually the latter'. It has also been argued that EE is no more than an indicator of stress and that the family interventions work because they do provide some support and advice which reduces that stress (Hatfield 1987a; Hatfield, Spaniol and Zipple 1987).

(b) *Problem solving and other supportive interventions*

There are other approaches which do not take a theoretical perspective on families, but do offer a variety of supportive programmes (Solomon et al. 1997). An example of a well-publicized approach is that described in Falloon and Fadden (1993). Their programme entails a team of mental health professionals working with families in the community in a very pragmatic way. They set up goal-orientated programmes and interventions that revolve around the idea of problem solving. Whilst these approaches may well be important in providing valuable support to families, they have not been producing insight into the experiences of families.

2.1.3 Burden Research

Following Grad and Sainsbury's (1963) conceptualization, 'burden research' is a body of work which has sought to describe, or measure, the effects of mental illness on the family. According to Lefley (1997), there are now at least 21 instruments to measure the burden on families in cases of severe mental illness. This work can be seen as reactive to a lot of the family therapy work. It takes the view that a mentally ill person is a burden inflicted upon the family. This is really the contrary view of the early family therapists. It asks the question: what ill effects are caused in the family members, by the mentally ill person?

Stephen Platt reviewed this work in 1985 and drew particular attention to the distinction made between objective and subjective burden (Platt 1985). Objective burden involves practical matters, anything that occurs as an obviously disrupting factor in family life owing to the patient's condition (Winefield and Harvey 1994 provide a particularly clear example). This can be anything from financial effects to the disruption of routines and of previous roles. These elements are generally easily measurable, almost by definition, in that they involve perceived burden or difficulties. Subjective burden involves the feelings engendered by the objective burdens. The measurement of subjective burden is considered to be problematic (Platt 1985; Tarrier 1996), since the very subjectivity of the data presents difficulties for quantitatively orientated research. This subjective burden is, however, crucial since this is how people actually experience and are affected by the objective burdens that are being catalogued (Pickett et al. 1997). Apparently similar 'burdens' will mean different things to different people in different contexts (Greenberg, Kim and Greenley 1997). Researchers have begun, for example, to draw attention to the different perceptions of burden within different ethnic groups (Jenkins and Schumacher 1999; Stueve, Vine and Strueng 1997; Wong 2000). This emphasizes how important it is to understand more fully the perspectives of the individual family members – a concern that informs the rest of this book.

Objective measures of stress

Some studies have documented the stress suffered by relatives, using objective measures of illness and stress. Studies published by *The Scottish Schizophrenia Research Group* (1987) are a particularly clear example of this approach. They use self-report questionnaires (the 'General Health Questionnaire' and the 'Social Adjustment Scale') which they administer to relatives. They demonstrated very high levels of stress, with anxiety-based symptoms being prominent (see also Brown and Birtwhistle 1998 for a longitudinal study of the impact on families). Recognition of the strain and burden borne by families has led to some interest in the United States in respite care for families (Zirul, Lieberman and Rapp 1989). Researchers working in this area are not attempting to provide insight into the experience of relatives, they are satisfied simply to document the apparent toll on relatives.

2.1.4 The Exploratory Studies

A relatively small body of work, which has attempted to explore the perspective of the families, has noted the high levels of distress that families experience and the poor relationships that seem to exist between professionals and families.

Perring, Twigg and Atkin (1990), in lamenting the dearth of studies that examine what it is actually like to care for someone with serious mental illness, argue that the paucity of such research might partly be explained by the strong medical bias that has guided research in this area. This has meant the experience of people (particularly those not actually 'ill') has been ignored in the quest for 'cure', and through medical science's reliance on quantitative methods. Studies of families where there is mental illness present, which do not attempt to identify the cause – or alter the course – of mental illness were, until very recently, very few and far between. Two sociological studies carried out in the 1950s made some interesting observations (Clausen and Yarrow 1954; Mills 1962).

American sociologists Clausen and Yarrow (1954) looked at the wives of people suffering mental illness. The perspective taken by the study was actually quite a traditional medical model. It was concerned with examining how mental illness came to be recognized as such by the family members. Its conclusions are about how public education might quicken this recognition and thus make families request medical help sooner.

British sociologist Enid Mills (1962) carried out a study of mental illness in the late 1950s in the East End of London. She documents some of the hardship and suffering endured by families, and comments on the apparently very involved, close relationships that seem to develop, particularly between mothers and sons who are ill. This observation is similar to some of those made at this time by the American family therapists who assumed that those mothers were causing the problems. Mills also noted the often poor relationships between GPs and relatives, with relatives feeling bitter that illness was not recognized or treated properly. This finding is echoed in later studies by Creer (1975), Holden and Lewine (1982), Shepherd, Murray and Muijen (1994) and Strong (1997), which all highlight the often poor relationships that families seem to have with service agencies and professionals. As should be clear by now, given the policy ambivalence and some of the theories informing professionals' attitudes, these findings may not be surprising.

Clare Creer (1975) has provided certainly the best known, and probably most in-depth, look at the problems faced by relatives in the UK. She carried out a survey of informal carers who had been involved in the formation of the National Schizophrenia Fellowship (NSF). She interviewed 50 NSF members and also 30 non-NSF relatives in an attempt to counterbalance the self-selectivity of the NSF sample. Various data were collected on the characteristics of the patient. More data were collected on the feelings and difficulties faced by the relatives themselves. She uncovered a great deal of distress: 47.5 per cent of the sample described their health or well-being as being impaired to a 'severe' or 'very severe' extent; only 18.8 per cent described their health or well-being as not being impaired. Much of the stress was caused by the unpredictable behaviour of the cared-for person.

Creer's sample levelled a great deal of criticism at the services that were available. Relatives also often felt that help had not been available until late in the day, when traumatic compulsory hospital admission would occur. Following discharge there would be little in the way of support. Creer also describes anxiety and depression as being reactions to the difficult and traumatic circumstances faced by the relative. In addition, grief was experienced, because relatives felt that the person they had once known had 'gone away'. This grief was exacerbated, as relatives often felt that professionals made no attempt to understand this. Indeed it was felt that professional workers judged relatives as being 'over-anxious' or 'unstable', sometimes even explicitly blaming them for causing the illness.

A small study, consisting of guided interviews with ten relatives of people on a Community Psychiatric Nursing case-load, is reported by Simmons (1990). Simmons describes her work as 'illuminative research' and, indeed, the study includes some very interesting quotations and discussions, which might well provide insight into the experiences of these ten people. There is little analysis of those experiences, so that the conclusion consists essentially of two points: firstly, that families need more information, and, secondly, that professionals should take more notice of what families say and that what is required of professionals is a more collaborative approach.

Mona Wasow (1995) uses her own experiences of coping with her son's serious mental illness to inform research interviews with siblings, children, grandparents and other extended family members. This book represents a valuable step forward in highlighting the misery and pain suffered by families. A couple of the themes that emerge from that book, particularly the emphasis on the grief process, will be picked up later in this book. Victoria Secunda (1997) has produced a more journalistic book that includes some valuable material and observations. There is a literature emerging from the United States, which Cook, Pickett and Cohler (1997: 172) have termed 'the next generation of research', that has been influenced by the family consumer movement (Hatfield 1987b) and the voices of personal experience.[1] The thrust of this literature is to encourage much more sympathetic consideration of the needs of the families. Some of the issues picked up by this literature will be taken up in the following chapters.

Families' experiences: what do we need to know?

A review of the published research on families and serious mental illness reveals a great volume of research. It is, however, work that tells us little about the experiences of those families. The majority of the

---

[1] Lanquetot (1988) and Willis (1982) are good examples of 'first-person accounts' from the journal *Schizophrenia Bulletin*.

studies have approached families with specific ideological biases that
have made understanding hard to achieve. They have tended to objectify family members, which has made understanding their subjective
states problematic. In 1987 Terkelsen (1987: 129) was able to comment,
in reviewing the area for a book chapter, 'so few formal studies of the
meaning of mental illness exist that this chapter could be a catalog of
required rather than completed research'. It becomes clear that fresh
research is necessary to build on the findings of the small number of
exploratory studies. The rest of the chapter will outline the methodology for a study of people who have a close relative who falls into the
category of 'new long-stay' (who represent the real challenge to those
seeking alternatives to the asylums, as discussed in the Introduction).
The findings of this study form the bases of the subsequent chapters.

2.2 Methodology for the Exploration of the Experiences of Relatives

In-depth, relatively unstructured, interviews were the chosen method
of investigation. There are two major methodological strands to the
study. Firstly, I wanted to try and understand the perspectives and
experiences of the families. In this I was influenced by a strong tradition
of phenomenologically informed qualitative research in sociology (Bittner
1973; Bleicher 1982; Bogdan and Taylor 1975; Glaser and Strauss 1967;
Rogers 1983; Schutz 1954, 1967; Silverman 1985, 1993; Strauss 1987).
There has also been a more recent growth in interest in such work in
psychology (Harré 1981; Hollway 1989; Potter and Wetherell 1987; and
Smith, Jarman and Osborn 1999). Despite the long history of qualitative
work, there have been well-recorded difficulties with incorporating the
study of emotional worlds of individuals (Craib 1995; Johnson 1975;
Kleinman and Copp 1993; Oakley 1981; O'Connell Davidson and Laydor
1994; Scully 1990). Since I was particularly interested in examining the
emotional impacts and understandings of events, it was also necessary
to utilize ideas with roots in psychodynamic thought (Hunt 1989).
Simply put, this was an understanding that a research interview is an
event that entails communications occurring at covert and emotional
levels (see Casement 1985, 1989 and Malan 1979 for discussions of
theory and technique, and Klauber 1981 for methodological discussion
of psychoanalysis).

A weakness of the reliance on interviews is that it provides only
cross-sectional 'snapshots' of situations where there are good reasons
to believe that they have been evolving for many years. This inadequacy,

however, could at least be acknowledged and taken into account. Indeed, relevant periods for some people covered over 30 years, so longitudinal study would simply not have been practicable. Observational techniques could also have less easily coped with this historical aspect. Interviews have long been used to gather biographical data or 'life histories', where the assumption is that people can only be understood within the context of their histories (Bertaux 1981, for example).

The aim of the style of interviewing was to provide space for the relatives' story to be heard, and for their understanding of that story to emerge. The chief framework for the interviews was provided by the context of the research. I was a researcher, connected to the health authority, who was trying to understand the interviewees' experiences of having a relative suffer from severe mental health difficulties. I emphasized through the introductory letter, and what I said when we met, that I was there to listen to what they had to say. This message was reinforced by what I tried to communicate throughout the interview. I used a tape-recorder whenever possible, so I could concentrate on listening. I provided a framework for the interviews by having certain questions in my mind:

- What does this person understand about what has happened? What does it mean to them?
- What sort of relationship do they have with the ill person? What does the relationship mean?
- What sort of relationship do they have with the health and social services? What do they think of the treatments that have been offered?
- How does what has happened affect their lives?
- Does what has happened affect their relationships with others? Is there stigma involved?

Most of these questions were implied by the context of the interview and were therefore addressed spontaneously by the interviewees. I would find ways of asking those questions that did not arise naturally. Interestingly, the questions about stigma were ones that I most often had to raise (the significance of stigma and shame is discussed in detail in Chapter 6).

The details of the sample are described in Appendices A and B. It is important to note that the definition of family used was entirely loose. Once a group of people who could be described as fitting into the category of 'new long-stay' was identified, anyone who could be contacted and agreed to be interviewed was interviewed. The interview sample was not confined to people who shared a household (the vast majority did not), nor to particular familial relations.

2.2.1 Ethnicity

The sample was drawn from a highly multicultural area of North London. Given the over-representation of Afro-Caribbeans amongst users of psychiatric services (King et al. 1994), it not surprising that 17 of the 34 sample families can broadly be described as Afro-Caribbean.

As will become clear in the following chapters, the interviews were not analysed systematically in terms of ethnicity. This is due to the substantial problems with analyses along cultural and ethnic lines (see Lambert and Sevak 1996 and Ahmad 1996 for powerful critiques of studies of cultural and ethnic difference in health). Certainly, ethnicity and social class are highly complex and multifaceted phenomena. Within the category 'Afro-Caribbean' there were people with roots as diversely placed as Nigeria, South Africa, Jamaica and Barbados. To have allotted people to rigid groupings would have been quite at odds with the approach I have taken: which is, in significant part, an attempt to analyse what lies underneath common-sense categories.

As detailed in Appendix A, however, four out of the five families who refused to be recorded were Afro-Caribbean. This is very likely to reflect something important about the feelings of alienation from psychiatric services amongst ethnic minorities (Fernando 1991; Littlewood and Lipsedge 1989).

2.2.2 Gender

A systematic analysis of gender differences is perhaps the most surprising omission. A great deal of literature on caring has emphasized the disproportionate amount of caring that is carried out by women (Ungerson 1990). The distinction that has been made between 'caring for' and 'caring about someone' (Mason 1994) is perhaps relevant here. This book is less concerned with the labour of caring than with the feelings involved. The fact that I was generally interviewing people who were not living together meant that the notion of caring was not merely confined to the domestic. As will become clear in the following chapters, the pain endured and talked about by men was often great and not obviously distinguishable from that experienced by women. This is confirmed by Davis and Schultz's (1997) attempt to quantify the depth of grief experienced by parents of people suffering from schizophrenia, where they found no differences between mothers and fathers.

The fact that I interviewed more women than men (see Appendix B) is probably the most significant point about gender, with women being more involved in family relationships and more willing to talk about them (Duncombe and Marsden 1993; Finch and Groves 1984; Oakley 1981).

2.2.3 Presentation of the Interview Material

There is a seeming contradiction in the aims of the study. On the one hand, I was interested in providing a platform for the voices of an under-represented group to be heard (Berger Gluck and Patai 1991; Oakley 1981). On the other, I was looking underneath the words that the interviewees used (Smith, Jarman and Osborn 1999). I am offering *my* interpretations of what they say. They are undoubtedly highly subjective explorations. The findings are presented in such a way as to try and make that process as transparent as possible. The interview material presented in the following sections is annotated. All the inter- view material is preceded by text which contains numbered points referring to places within the transcript; these are my reflections on what is being said. This is an attempt to expose the process of analysis as much as possible and to still allow the voices of the families to be heard. In addition, I have made liberal use of the first person, in part to reinforce that these are not simply objective facts (Richardson 1990), but are my attempts to make sense of what people said to me.

In the following material all names have been changed and all ident- ities have been disguised.

3

The Complicated Grief: 'Living on the edge of the world'

The analysis of the families' experiences will begin with their grief. The significance of grief has been strongly emphasized by those who have looked at the impact of mental illness on families (Creer 1975; Davis and Shultz 1997; Lanquetot 1988; MacGreggor 1994; Spaniol, Zipple and Lockwood 1992; Wasow 1995). As the first section of this chapter will describe, this grief is triggered by the apparently universal perception that there was a very marked discontinuity in the behaviour and being of their relative. It is important to note that this discontinuity was invariably seen as a negative change and that a broadly medical explanation was assumed. This aspect of the families' experience is important. For all the various ways of understanding mental distress – whether as organic disease, as psychological disorder, social construct or as intolerance of deviance – this is how this group perceived their relatives' difficulties.

As many writers have noted, grief can be regarded as a process (Freud 1917; Marris 1978; Murray Parkes 1972). Murray Parkes, in his classic study of bereavement (1972), writes explicitly about the stages of grief as a natural process, consisting roughly of a phase of denial, followed by one of protest, followed by one of acceptance. Much of the writing about grief has been in a similar vein, highlighting cases where the pathway through the process has become complicated (Kubler-Ross 1973; Littlewood 1992; Wertheimer 1991). The case will be made here for understanding these relatives' experiences in terms of a process of grieving that is not easy to navigate. Atkinson (1994) highlights the tendency towards 'chronic grieving' in families coping with serious mental illness. Willick (1994), for example, has described his own feelings as a father of a man diagnosed as suffering from schizophrenia as a 'mourning without end'.

A number of suggestions have been put forward to explain this pattern of chronic grief. MacGregor (1994) suggests that this is an example

of 'disenfranchised grief', meaning that people feel unable to communicate their grief since this loss is not understood or acknowledged by
others and the shame of mental illness may inhibit people from talking
about their experiences. Certainly the presence of good social support
networks has been identified as an important factor in helping people
through the process of grief (Littlewood 1992). It has also been suggested that this grief is more difficult to resolve than loss through death
because the families are constantly reminded of their loss (MacGregor
1994; Willick 1994). The second section of this chapter will explore this
experience of chronic grief. It will be argued that these relatives' grief is
made difficult by the particular circumstances that they typically face,
which can lead to powerful feelings of ambivalence both towards the
person who suffers from the mental illness and towards the process that
might lead to a resolution of that grief. As Freud (1917) and subsequent
writers have noted, the bereaved person has to accommodate not only
to the loss of the past, but also to the loss of future expectations – the
events and experiences they might have shared with the person who has
gone. This latter loss is particularly poignant for those who feel they
have 'lost' someone to mental illness because their relatives are still
around, however much altered.

3.1   The Experience of Discontinuity

Although the perception of change was universal there were differences
in the way this change was seen. Four categories can usefully be distinguished. One group reported an abrupt realization that their relative
had changed very suddenly. A second group recounted that they had
more gradually realized that their relative had changed. A third group
felt their relative, although having reached a crisis and a point of abrupt
change, had perhaps always been a bit different. A fourth group described
observing their relative as being in a process of gradual deterioration. It
may well be that these retrospective accounts do reflect real differences
in the rates of onset of their relatives' difficulties.

One example should suffice here to illustrate a few points about
change and some assumptions that were made about that change. Elly
Blacksmith, now in her seventies, was herself born in Jamaica but has
brought up her family in London. Her response is typical of those who
reported a sudden realization of an abrupt change in her son, who now
has a diagnosis of schizophrenia and lives nearby in a council flat. He
goes around most days and helps his mother with routine household

chores. This seemed to be what could be described as a very 'reconciled' situation (discussed in Chapter 8, pp. 147–50).

In response to the opening question, Mrs Blacksmith refers back to an event occurring at a specific time – indeed, a certain date has stuck in Mrs Blacksmith's memory (1). The time is associated with an exam, which perhaps marks a point of development and achievement (that has not been maintained). A hypothesis of cause is hinted at: 'studying a bit too hard' (3). All these issues are important and will be returned to in later chapters. Previously, Mrs Blacksmith had noticed that he was behaving slightly oddly: 'speaking a lot of different stupidness' (2). It is, however, a very public display of remarkable behaviour (a crowd gathers, as her son takes off his clothes (4)) occurring alongside a violent incident (he threatens to harm himself with a meat cleaver) which brings matters to full recognition. Mrs Blacksmith's response to this crisis is to call the doctor (5). It is noteworthy (and, as we shall see, this is a common belief) that apparently very straightforwardly the aberrant behaviour is construed as a medical problem. Mrs Blacksmith presents her perception of a pattern of events (6). The pattern is seen as being a cyclical one of illness (7). The illness is described in terms that are compatible with a psychiatric construction: 'From there every year, or every two year probably, he gets a breakdown' (6). The breakdown follows a pattern of 'depression' followed by 'withdrawal' and then him doing 'stupid things'.

EB: Well, you ask the questions . . .
DJ: When did you first notice things going wrong?
EB: It was in 1980 [1] when he was supposed to take his exams he was supposed to sit for his City and Guilds . . . and then it was on the 8th, he was supposed to take his exams on the 13th, and then on the 8th he started to go a bit funny, speaking a lot of different stupidness [2]. He was studying a bit hard really [3] to sit for his exams and then . . . I was living in Cornell Road and then once a crowd gathered, I had a friend living in this area she saw the crowd and when she went up she saw that it was my son taking off all his clothes [4]. She put him in a taxi and fetch him home . . . no first he went into a butcher shop and took out the meat thing, cleaver or whatever it is, to . . . you know chop up himself and she brought him home. I called the private doctor [5], the doctor came and recommend him to the hospital. From there every year, or every two year probably, he gets a breakdown [6]. But you notice what he does – he goes into a right depression state first and kind of withdrawal after that, you can

see, because you see the stupid things sometimes. When he
smoke his cigarettes, he buy a packet of ten he would put all in
the fingers and then smoke them one after the other [demon-
strates putting a cigarette in between all fingers] from that you
get to know each time he's taking ill [7].

3.1.1   Distress Objectified and Medicalized

Mrs Blacksmith is typical in her perception that some *thing* had happened
to her son. There is perceived to be a very definite rupture with past
behaviour. As already mentioned, some families do not always report
such a definite point in time, some saying, for example, that they became
aware of change more gradually. All the families shared the view that
some *thing* had happened to their relative. This thing, most usually considered to be 'an illness', has either emerged from within their family
member, or has been inflicted on them from the outside world. The
details of how this has come about will be discussed in the following
chapters. The important point to note is that the 'it' is seen as being
separate from the true self of the relative. It may be covering up, or it
may have usurped this true self. It will become clearer in the following
section that this model does bring considerable psychological benefits
in helping families accept the often difficult behaviour of their ill relative (Kinsella, Anderson and Anderson 1996).

Alongside the perception of something happening to change their
relative was an apparently automatic and easy decision that this was a
medical problem. Mrs Blacksmith is typical in reporting that her first
response to the perception of a problem was to call the doctor. In many
ways, the relatives' constructions of what has happened are consistent
with the mainstream psychiatric picture of illness. This raises the possibility, as other authors have suggested (Perelberg 1983a), that the
families have simply learnt, or have introjected, the psychiatric model
from professionals they have had contact with. It will be argued in the
following chapters that this is probably too simplistic. As the next chapter will explore, the families seemed often to hold quite sceptical attitudes towards professionals and their theories and were quite active
themselves in appropriating psychiatric terms for their own use.

3.1.2   Diminishment

Perhaps not surprising, although still worth mentioning because it has
great implications for the emotional impact on relatives, is the fact that

the change that had occurred is seen in negative terms, as a diminishment. This change is one that brings a great deal of pain. Where positive aspects of people's personalities were seen to exist, this was usually *in spite of* illness. Instances of positive elements being associated with the illness itself were very rare. Mr Doors, for example, did see within his daughter a certain heightened awareness of the 'spiritual' nature of life that was associated with her illness. Jean Karajac associated his sister's illness with her being a very perceptive person. In the main the perception was that something had happened to their relative and that this was experienced as a loss. The next section will examine this experience of change in terms of loss and as a complex grief reaction.

3.2   An Exploration of Complex Grief: the Problem of Ambivalence

It will be argued that there are aspects of the particular circumstances of this group of relatives that will often mean that the pathway through grief is a convoluted one. One of the chief sources of difficulty are the feelings of ambivalence that are inspired both towards the person who is ill, and towards the idea of coming to an acceptance of the changes that they have witnessed.

Ambivalence has been emphasized as a major factor that interferes with the process of grief (Freud 1917; Marris 1978; Murray Parkes 1972). Marris (1978) argues that the whole grief process is marked by ambivalence, in that the bereaved person is torn between wanting to remain attached to that which is lost and wanting to move on from that and find meaning in the new circumstances. People who are bereaved will often express this quite directly: that they do not want to forget the person, that in going over memories, seeming to torture themselves with memories, they are deriving some comfort from remaining with the person. There is no denial of the reality of the loss. Instead there is denial of the possibility of carrying on without the lost person. According to Marris, bereavement is never straightforward. It is always a process that involves a struggle with mixed feelings. On the one hand, we do not like change, yet on the other, we know we must adapt and accommodate to change in order to carry on. Two further sources of ambivalence can be identified that were prominent in these families' experiences.

(1)   *Hostile feelings.*   The behaviour of someone with serious mental health problems is often unpredictable and will often invoke feelings of anger and hostility (Creer 1975; Wasow 1995). These feelings,

it will be argued, can interfere with the process of grief (Murray Parkes 1972).

(2) ***The fear of betrayal.***   Although a loss has been experienced, it is, after all, only based on a perception of change. The person has not really gone away. On one level, this means constant visible reminders of loss (Brodoff 1988; Wasow 1995; Willick 1994). On another level, the bereavement is complicated by the fear of betraying the old person, if accommodation is made with the apparently different person that has emerged.

Both of these particular factors will now be examined in some detail.

3.2.1   Hostile and Mixed Feelings

Murray Parkes (1972) drew particular attention to situations in which people had ambivalent, or sometimes frankly hostile, feelings towards someone before they died. Subsequent grief is then complicated by the ensuing feelings of guilt. One particular aspect of the ambivalent mourning of the relatives interviewed here is that they are likely currently to harbour some hostile feelings towards the ill person. They have to endure guilt, not only about feelings they had in the past, but their current negative feelings.

Anger itself is a seemingly common, perhaps ubiquitous, reaction to grief through loss or change. Bowlby (1980), using the theoretical framework of Melanie Klein (Klein 1946; Steiner 1992), argued that this anger has its roots in an infant's protest at felt neglect, demanding of the mother's attention, and is therefore a normal aspect of grief (Murray Parkes 1972). As the infant develops and gains a better understanding of the world, this anger becomes associated with anxiety and guilt since the stimulant of the anger is also that which is most loved and valued. The cases studied here are particularly beset with ambivalence. The most obvious source of the anger is the ill person. However, this is someone who is construed as being subject to an illness, and therefore as deserving of sympathy. Nevertheless, the ill person has also brought pain; pain through simply becoming something different, and pain from the ensuing traumatic and dramatic events (MacGregor 1994). The difficulty of what to do with those feelings of anger is amplified.

Despite the fact that anger did seem to be commonly present, we will see in later chapters how assiduously family members would protect their relatives from direct blame. Anger directed towards someone who suffers from mental illness seems illegitimate. Wertheimer (1991: 172) noted a similar problem amongst people whose relatives had committed suicide. They *were* angry, but felt this was an illegitimate feeling. To relatives of people with mental illness the biomedical model is useful because the illness itself provides a safe target for their anger. Kinsella, Anderson and Anderson suggest that this objectification of the illness is an important coping strategy. They quote a sibling's blunt advice: 'Separate the illness from the person and say it's alright to hate the illness and it's best to love the person' (Kinsella, Anderson and Anderson 1996: 27).

In the following extract I tried to clarify Fred Bryant's attitude to the long-stay hospital (Friern hospital) where his son was resident. His attitude had puzzled me. On the one hand, the hospital was described, with some disgust, as looking like 'something out of a horror movie'. On the other hand, he was angry about the Health Authority's plans to close that hospital. As discussed in the next chapter, there is perhaps an element of desperation here in that, whilst he does not like the hospital, he feels that it is a port in a storm. I do not think it is taking too much liberty with interpretation, however, to suggest that this particular ambivalence obscures some aggressive feelings towards his son. He would prefer him to jump in front of a tube train (1) than live his life in hospital. Fred feels that it is the families that suffer the most (2).

DJ: In the past people have spent their lives in Friern, would you want to see that for John?

FB: ... Well maybe, to be perfectly brutal about it, I'd prefer him to jump in front of a tube train [1] than spend his whole life from 22 to 69 or 70 locked away there. But Friern don't affect John, I don't think it affects a lot of them, it's the parents and the people that are helping that it drives... that sort of feel it [2]. A lot of these patients, it doesn't bother them. You know they don't seem to bother as much as the people that are worried about them.

Elsewhere in the interview Fred Bryant is asked about his own continuing involvement (this is a man who has made a remarkable sacrifice in that he gave up his home in the north of England to live with his son in London). He first of all mentions the fact of his relationship – 'he's my son' (1). The way that people made recourse to apparently common-sense notions of the importance of family is a theme that is fully developed in Chapter 7 ('The Myth of the Family'). There is also a confession of more negative feelings (2). As Fred Bryant continues to talk he mentions his own death (3) and then through further rumination there is an association to another patient who committed suicide (4).

DJ: What's made you be so involved? You said yourself before that a lot of families drop out, they can't cope any more, but you've kept going?

FB: Well I suppose... it's really because he's my son [1], and there are certainly times... when I just don't ever want to see him again [2]. There's certainly those times... It's like to really give you the answer to that, it's like I'm the only one there, there's no-one else for John, if I disappear that's it,... when I die [3] I sort of think that maybe my son Peter will step in, I think that quite possibly... he's a publisher. He's doing well. John's brother is a publisher and his sister is a business analyst, they're both up there and he's down there. But I think when – if I die I do think that Peter will step in... to some extent, not to the same extent as I have done, but I think he will step in to some extent, I don't know... I just think that will possibly happen, knowing the nature of him. But it is hard, I mean I know other parents that go there, the problems that they have, you see the amount of people there that just don't get anybody at all. One particular instance a woman called Pat, I think, she had an outside job. She lived in ward 23, she jumped in front of a train and committed suicide [4].

Perhaps this rumination that shifts from his own death to the suicides of other sufferers suggests that Fred does wonder if his son's death would present a kind of resolution to what seems to be an intractable problem (one that he fears will continue after his death when he is powerless to help). The worry about 'what will become of them after my death' was frequently expressed during interviews and has been remarked upon elsewhere (Creer 1975; Lanquetot 1988). There are a number of ways of understanding this concern. As discussed further in Chapter 7, it can be argued that ideas about the continuity of family relationships are a way of seeing ourselves continuing beyond death (Bauman 1992; Borneman 1996; Bouquet 1996). For people to feel that their children are damaged by mental illness is a threat to this continuity. Erikson's (1963) notion that the final stage of later life involves the struggle between feelings of integrity versus despair may be another way of understanding this thinking. Erikson argued that for satisfactory mental health in older age it was essential to develop a feeling that what you have done, what you have built and created in your life, is valuable and worthwhile. The struggle is with the feeling of despair that what has been created is flawed or not worthwhile. Fred Bryant's talk of his own death suggests a concern with a review of his life, and what will happen when he has gone. The allusion to suicide implies dissatisfaction, that things are not as they should be, the world is not safe to let go of.

The reference to suicide may also suggest a degree of aggression. Fear of their relatives committing suicide was something that interviewees often brought up. Clearly it is a real fear and no doubt the grief they would feel would be great. I began, however, to see the repeated references to suicide as containing aggressive feelings. Wasow (1995: 116) has written bravely of her own 'dark thoughts' about her son, sometimes thinking 'that he'd be better off dead'. I was able to explore this notion over a couple of extended interviews with Jacob Doors. These thoughts, as Wasow says, are indeed dark, they are often hidden and are undoubtedly hard to express. It seems worthwhile to present their emergence during interviews in some detail, since this is how professionals working with families are most likely to come across them – not as fully expressed ideas but as hints of darker thoughts that professionals might need to take into account.

Jacob Doors made several references to his fears about his daughter, April, committing suicide. His response to my remarking on one of these references was to tell me that it is something he dreams about. This suggests an element of wish fulfilment. In his sleep he gets rid of his daughter (1), but wakes with feelings of guilt about how he should have done more for her. He then ruminates guiltily (2) on how busy he is as a businessman. In doing so he also allows himself to imagine how things might be if she were not around:

DJ: This is something that concerns you particularly, the risk of suicide?

JD: Yes, now that you mention it, yes, yes. It's a bit at the back of my mind now because she's taking the medication and she appears better, but it is, yes, it is a worry, yes. Mmm. It is a worry. Sometimes I wake up in a dream and think that it's happened [1] and I feel terrible about it. It doesn't happen very often but it does happen... I haven't got an awful lot of time for April [2], I've got my work, and if I don't work I won't eat, I'll sort of be bankrupt, [edit]... so I've got to keep going. But it does bother me. I wake up in these dreams 'Gosh I wish I'd spent more time with her' and things like that. It does bother me yes.... There you

are: ... So yes that is the main ... I think you've isolated the ...
what it's all about, that is the main worry at the bottom of it all.

Thus, it might be argued, the preoccupation with the risk of suicide
serves to allow Jacob Doors to have an aggressive 'fantasy' about his
daughter whilst the strong aggressive feelings he has are safely 'projected'
on to his daughter. The use of projection as a psychological mechanism
(Klein 1946) for coping with uncomfortable feelings is discussed further
in Chapter 6. Such dreams, or thoughts, allow someone to fantasize
about the demise of another and consider how life would be after their
relative's death.

A little later in the interview I feel brave enough to ask Jacob Doors
directly about aggressive feelings towards his daughter. He has no hesitation in agreeing (1). The two examples he gives are interesting, the
first to do with her own self-destructiveness (2), the second to do with
her breaking the 'sexual' boundaries in their relationship, as he suggests
she was jealous of the attention he pays to a young woman (3). It can be
argued that both of these produce aggression because they reveal
aspects of the relationship that are beset with ambivalence and are thus
difficult to manage. Both incidents challenge his authority, whilst
perhaps her own self-destructiveness accords too well with his own
aggressive feelings towards her, and the sexual boundary overstepped is
alarming within the context of the familial relationships. Perelberg
(1983a, 1983b) identified the breaching of sexual boundaries as being
an important factor in 'the accusation' of mental illness within families.
The importance of the observance of sexual boundaries will be
explored further in Chapter 7:

DJ: Do you sometimes get very angry with her?
JD: Yes, yes. Oh yes ... often in fact [1]. When she worked with me
     I'd be absolutely fuming, she'd do something, I don't know
     why ... it was quite irrational, other people said it was quite
     embarrassing, oh yes. ... yes definitely. I've hit her on a couple
     of occasions, just a clout around the ear on a couple of occa-
     sions. Happened ... she never believed in smoking and neither
     do I, one day she came in when she was 18, came back from the
     pub with her boyfriend, Greek boyfriend Tony who she was
     with. And she came in stinking of cigarettes, she'd been smoking
     [2]. And she says 'So what?', me spending all of my life talking
     to her about smoking, and her agreeing with me! And just to say
     'So what?' so cheekily, I felt my hand go 'wop wop' and it was

back by my side before I even thought. [edit]...The only other occasion I can think of [edit]...was again when she was a bit deranged. We went to Sainsbury's [supermarket] when I was a bachelor, as it were,...went to Sainsbury's and there was a girl there behind the counter and I started chattering to the cashier and I don't do that normally and on this occasion I did, she was about 20 I think. I said 'Oh you look like a French girl, like you see in French shops', which she did. 'Oh thank you, thanks a lot.' And April piped up 'He says that to all the girls!', making me look some dirty old man, I don't actually. That so annoyed me, and er she was doing that to spoil me chatting to the girl so I think [3]...and then she said something else when we got back to the car, and I was unloading the groceries and that was when my hand came up, she got a clout, before I reacted, she was clouted before I had time to think. The jealousy element, there might well be some truth in that, she might well have been jealous of me chatting up, she was trying to spoil my chances with that girl then. So there might well be some truth in it....Yes, I've been angry....She's got the ability to get me annoyed very, very quickly, I've got to control myself at all times.

In a second interview with Jacob Doors I felt able to go further and explore whether he ever actually thought he wanted his daughter to die. The question was framed very carefully:

DJ: Some families say, when things are really bad: 'Sometimes I wish they had taken that bottle of pills, they said they were going to take' – to kill themselves, things would be easier. Have you ever thought like that?

JD: Er...I'd say it has crossed my mind, yes. Don't think I've, I don't think I've verbalized it, even in my own head. But erm, yes it has, it has. I have thought about this, rather than the terrible wait, yep....I imagine people feel guilty about it as well....But it is a strain, and a strain is a strain, I mean I've made it less of a strain by just cutting myself off from April unless it's necessary – to the point of being abrupt, abrupt with her, you know sort of down to earth. It keeps a barrier between me and her and also, I like to think it helps her as well, rather than sort of moping. 'Oh dear I hope you don't hear those voices any more', I tend to be 'Oh well you're not on about that again are you!?' or 'Not this god lark!', you know and er...so

> I don't know. I think it might do it better. But yes I can under-
> stand someone thinking that, yes, yes.

This was a particularly reflective man who was able to think quite
deeply about his own feelings about his daughter. He may have been
unusual in his capacity for reflection – but perhaps not in having those
feelings. As many have noted, being a carer for someone with severe
mental health problems is a painful business (Creer 1975; Hatfield and
Lefley 1987; Mills 1962). The distress and resultant feelings of anger
are natural enough, but may well make any process of bereavement
more difficult.

3.2.2   The Fear of Betrayal

Whilst anger is very commonly present in grief it can be, as the above
example highlights, particularly poignant when someone is seen as
suffering from severe mental illness. There is another source of ambivalence that is perhaps more specific to this situation. We have seen
how people see their relatives as having fundamentally altered in an
important way. The ill person's 'self' is seen as having changed, or it is
covered over by illness, almost as though they have become someone
else. A fundamental discontinuity is experienced between the person
that was, with the person that has become. This, however, is not the
whole truth. In other ways the person is still around. Physically they
are not altered. There are very often signs, or even appearances, of the
old self still detectable (Creer 1975; Wasow 1995). Therefore another
aspect of the ambivalence in the bereavement studied here is the difficulty in reconciling the person that is lost with the person they have
become (Davis and Schultz 1997). This is a different, and perhaps
more difficult, process to negotiate than that associated with straightforward loss. In the latter the bereaved must come to terms with a new
situation that includes the absence of the lost person. Here there is the
apparent loss of a person accompanied by the emergence of a different
person.

   One woman who was able to offer particularly valuable insight into
the mourning process was Mrs Mansell, who has had experience as a
bereavement counsellor. She makes it clear what a difficult grieving
process is involved in accepting her husband's illness. She was separated from him at the time of the interviews but, since they shared a son,
contact persisted. She describes feeling that he uses something up
within her (1). However, she cannot move on from this because

although she knows she is grieving, that she has lost the person he was, he is not actually dead and she still has to see him (2):

DJ: How do you feel about Alfred now?

IM: Part of me has to see him sometimes. One thing is I can't grieve properly. If he had died you know what to do, being a bereavement counsellor, I know what to expect, what to do and you can perhaps make a new beginning, but with Alfred he's never asked me whether I have a relationship with anybody, I haven't, but he just takes it for granted that I'm here. I don't think I have anything left for another relationship [1].... If I see him, that shows me that he's not dead and that although I'm grieving (I know it's there it's true) I find it difficult to know that he's in the world, he's not dead [2] – Why's he not with us, because we'd like to be a normal family with a teenager, he's 14 in April. I would dearly love him to have daddy – but acknowledging that daddy couldn't cope anyway, the rest of me can do without that.

The ambivalence of grief is therefore doubly reinforced. To move on from the grief is not only difficult because it involves a betrayal of the memories of the past (as in 'normal' grief), but is difficult because the person is still around, however much altered. Brodoff (1988: 116) describes her feelings about her mentally ill brother when she spends time with him: 'I've missed my older brother with the persistent ache and longing usually reserved for a loved one lost through death.... However, mourning for a loved one who is alive – in your very presence and yet in vital ways inaccessible to you – has a lonely, unreal quality that is extraordinarily painful.'

Mrs Christian was a mother who was very conspicuously caught in the middle of traumatic grief. I met her several times, with a gap of two years between two recorded interviews. The interviews were in many ways very similar. She was highly involved with her son and his condition seemed to dominate her life. She visited him in hospital every other day. During both interviews she became tearful. Her feelings about her son and what had happened to him were clearly very painful. Twenty-five years on from his initial hospitalization and diagnosis, she seemed to be still traumatized and grief-stricken. I believe that this can be understood in terms of her reluctance to let go of the hopes and love she had for the person that he had been. For her, to do so would feel like a betrayal of that person.

Mrs Christian spoke warmly of her and her late husband's family, and she saw a great deal of a wider kin network. In spite of this, it seemed as though Mrs Christian felt that her experience with her son had left her feeling isolated within that family. She felt that her experiences could not be understood by others. She gained a great deal of support from her local National Schizophrenia Fellowship (NSF) branch, where she meets those who have had similar experiences. When she is asked about what support she gets, her first point of reference is her relatives (1). Neither families nor friends, however, can really understand what it is like; there is a gulf of understanding (2) in that she feels that people expect her to have got over the bereavement (her 40-year-old son having been diagnosed 25 years ago). She then goes on to describe what happened to her as something that is 'crippling' (3). This very direct appellation of her own distress is, however, then amended and effectively displaced from her. Mrs Christian recasts the description – the pain is then depicted as coming from 'watching' her son suffer from 'a crippling illness' (4). Within that couple of sentences, there seems to be an important truth about these relatives' experiences. I would suggest that Mrs Christian does feel *herself* to have been crippled by what has happened to her son. Like Mr Doors, above, it would be quite understandable if she harboured some quite angry feelings. She, however, feels guilt at reporting the damage that her son has done to her, whilst she still sees him as continuing to suffer. To seek to diminish her own pain would be as though she were 'turning [her] back on' her son (5). As Marris (1978) has suggested, ambivalence is at the core of the bereavement process. The central ambivalence of this grieving procss is that to move on and live life would feel like a betrayal, not just of a memory (in the case of loss through death) but of a person who is still very much around and suffering:

DJ: Do you have people you can turn to?
LC: Yes. I have lots of relatives [1] . . . I think sometimes they think, relatives and friends, that you should be used to it now [2]. I feel that's what they think, but you don't get used to it, how do you get used to such a crippling [3] . . . watching someone suffering from such a crippling illness [4]. It's not on . . . it would be turning your back on them [5]. You can sometimes stand back, and I do, you know try and be objective, there's still the pain and the hurt is there. . . .

As I wondered aloud about the isolation she feels, Mrs Christian's response suggests that this is a factor that makes it hard for her to negotiate her way through the grief process. Although her family are described as 'good and concerned' (1), there is revealing reference to their (and her own) appreciation of Peter in the past tense (2, 3, 4 and underlined). Mrs Christian jumps to talking about how Peter was some 20-odd years earlier when he was at school (5). What might be being expressed here is how difficult it is for Mrs Christian to reconcile those memories of her son as a successful schoolboy with the experience of him as he is now. This is an ongoing conflict, not open to easy reconciliation; 'I don't think you can ever get used to it' (6). Mrs Christian then uses a startling phrase, that she feels as though she is 'on the edge of the world' (8). Through this perturbing metaphor Mrs Christian gives voice to the feeling that her experience has isolated her; that, as others cannot comprehend her experience, she is left feeling excluded, on the edge of the discourse of the wider community. It is towards the fellow members of the NSF that she turns for comfort (7). It is there that she finds some common understanding of the long-term nature of the conflict. There is more consideration given in Chapter 6 to both the phenomenon, and the implications, of people finding comfort and solidarity within groups of families similarly affected.

DJ: Is it something you find difficult to talk about to people, because they don't understand?

LC: Sometimes yes. My sisters are very good and very concerned about Peter [1], he was loved by all my family [2], he was such a pleasant child [3]. He was never moody [4], never had problems with him... from an early age when he had homework he'd come home and start straight away [5]. My family do care. Some relatives, I find, think I should be used to it. I don't think you can ever get used to it [6], and a lot of our members [of the NSF] [7], if you really talk to them, they would say that you just learn to cope with the rest of the family or for each other, you learn to cope, that's all you do. You're living on the edge of the world sometimes [8], but people find it very hard, I think, to know how I'm feeling, I don't wear my heart on my sleeve. I tend to say 'I'm OK'.

Mrs Christian goes on to make comparison with Tom, a cousin of her son, who had become a lawyer and a journalist (1). Mrs Christian seems to struggle with anxiety about the fact that her son is not valued in ways that both he and she had perhaps hoped that he would be (through the early success in school).

Peter would ask me 'How's Tom doing?'. In the early days I found it hard to tell him that he's a journalist and a lawyer, doing very well [1]. Peter would say 'He must be very clever', I'd say 'Well, average, he works hard for it'. Peter has this thing on his locker on the ward, something like 'I am a genius I have a high IQ, if you don't believe me, ask the staff', he used to have it in the hostel as well. I said to him once, trying to get a reaction from him, 'Peter you're not living up to what it says on there, you could do lots of things, you could help yourself more, make life a lot easier for yourself' – 'I suppose so' he said. 'Why do you put it up there Peter, we all know you're clever anyway'. He said 'I want people to think that I am a some-body, I'm not a nobody'. I said: 'Of course Peter you're important, very important, don't ever forget it. You are a very important person to yourself, to me, to all the people you know.' It's very sad that he thinks that.

Hearing the contrast with the bold and angry statement of her son's worth at the end of that passage ('Peter you're important, very import-ant, don't ever forget it') and the former exclusive references to early success, prompted me to ask about what he means to her now (1). I think her response is no exaggeration (2), there seems little doubt that the situation dominates her life. Again, there are echoes of Erikson's description of the struggle of integrity versus despair (1963, 1982). Mrs Christian suggests that it dominates because she feels that she has to cope on her own. Mrs Christian would surely find MacGregor's (1994: 164) description of such as situation as 'disenfranchised grief' apt here. MacGregor suggests it is disenfranchised 'because society does not recognize and validate the existence or importance of the relationship, the loss, or the griever'. To Mrs Christian, professionals have failed and family do not fully understand. Only with fellow members of the NSF is there a chance of comfort through some common understanding:

DJ: What does Peter mean to you? [1]
LC: Everything really [2] ... I will always fight for Peter, as he's not able to do it himself. I don't care who I upset along the way, I shouldn't have to do this ... [becomes tearful] ... it should have just been there, 'Yes we'll try and help him, or find a suitable place for him'. If I was pushed, I would take it to the European courts. The Fellowship have been absolutely fantastic, ... you never have to explain to them how you feel, they know exactly how it feels.

3.3 Summary

These relatives' experiences must be understood in terms of a bereavement process. It is, however, a highly complicated bereavement. Whilst
the commonly considered bereavement processes that accompany loss
can be seen as being beset with ambivalence, as Marris (1978) has
argued, the process in this case is peculiarly prone to ambivalence
because:

(1) Anger is likely to be a strong feature of their experience, and they
     are likely to feel anger towards the person whom they also feel to
     be ill and therefore deserving of sympathy.
(2) Alongside the loss of the old person there is the experience of
     a new person to accommodate to. There is a fear of betraying the
     'old' person.

There seems little doubt that this process of bereavement is a key one.
There are yet further complicating factors that will be considered in the
following chapters. Other writers on grief have emphasized that pain is
derived not only from the loss of the past but also from the loss of
future possibilities (Freud 1917). This issue is dealt with in Chapter 7.
The next chapter will begin to explore the apparently ambivalent relationship that these relatives have with the psychiatric and medical professionals that they had contact with. Chapter 5 will examine families'
ideas about the causes of mental illness and Chapter 6 will examine the
influence of the stigmatizing status of mental illness on the relatives.
The point that should come across very strongly is that the process
involved in the navigation through the bereavement process does not
simply proceed in isolation, but involves an engagement with the wider
community as continuity of meaning must be found. Wertheimer (1991)
studied the experiences of people who have lost relatives through suicide. She describes how people were very positively helped in their grief
by realizing that other people loved and valued the person that had
been lost. Thus comfort was drawn from the finding that their distress
and their understanding of what has happened has a coherence and
value within the discourse around them. Unfortunately for the relatives
who feel they have lost someone to mental illness, the experience of
stigma and the feelings of shame that are associated with mental illness,
and the poor relationships with professionals, were often impediments
to engagement with the discourse of the wider community. As Mrs
Christian put it so effectively, she feels 'on the edge of the world'. The

issue of the relationship that families reported with professionals, and the lack of comfort or reassurance they gathered from them will be explored in the following chapter. This issue is important because the poor relationship that families often seem to have with professionals might seem odd, given (as this chapter has highlighted) that they both hold the essentials of an illness model to explain their relatives' difficulties.

4

The Relationship with Psychiatry and Psychiatric Knowledge

Critics working in the tradition of 'anti-psychiatry' (most famously Szasz 1970 in the United States, Laing 1959 in Britain) would suggest that the fact that relatives applied an illness model is a result of the dominance of psychiatric thought, which is itself a symptom of the medicalization of Western society (Illich 1977). Simply put, aspects of human experience connected perhaps to unhappiness, deviance or protest are neutralized and marginalized by being understood within medical and psychiatric frameworks. However, other work in medical sociology has suggested that professionals are not acting alone in the process of diagnosis but that 'others, including the patients themselves, are full participants in the process of labelling, diagnosis, management and treatment of illness' (Mishler 1981: 166). This latter view is consistent with the argument being made here that the relatives themselves are important actors in defining mental illness.

The next chapter ('The Moral Construction of Diagnosis') will explore, in detail, the theories about illness that people held. This chapter will examine what the relatives had to say about their relationship with mental health professionals and the services provided by them. The first section will note that specific diagnostic categories were regarded with some scepticism, and even when people talked about definite diagnoses the understanding of what that meant was often quite a limited, popular idea of mental illness (such as schizophrenia meaning 'split personality'). The second section will examine what the families had to say about their relationship to professionals. The relationships seemed to be characterized by hostility and suspicion. Families often felt that professionals, far from forcing labels onto people, were withholding information, and diagnoses in particular. Some of the conflict between professionals and families can be understood in terms of a dispute over the control of information. The third section will explore the families' view of the treatments that were made available. In fact, although the families very often construed their relatives' difficulties in medical terms, they seemed to have limited faith in the treatments and service provisions that were available.

4.1   The Meaning of Diagnosis

It was noticeable that formal diagnoses were rarely spontaneously mentioned during interviews. It did not seem as though the formal diagnosis was considered to be particularly meaningful. Mr and Mrs Rivers were an example of people who seemed to have extremely little formal knowledge. Their daughter had very clearly been diagnosed as suffering from schizophrenia. They did not seem to be aware of this, certainly the word was not mentioned during the interview, even after some prompting. During the interview, when asked what they thought was wrong, they focused on her unusual hand-washing, linking this to sickness, having seen something on television about this (presumably about obsessional hand-washing). Despite having very little psychiatric knowledge, they did not doubt that their daughter was 'sick'.

It was more usual for people to have been informed of a diagnosis, at some point. This did not, however, usually seem to carry very much meaning. For example, during the interview with Liz Regan and her husband, concerning their views on her sister's illness, no mention was made about any diagnosis until they were asked. It seemed that they had been asking professionals for information and eventually had been told that Liz's sister had been given a diagnosis of 'schizophrenia'. This did not, however, seem to mean a great deal to them. When asked what the diagnosis of schizophrenia meant to them, there is a hint that they hold the popular view as meaning 'split personality' (1), even though their observations of the behaviours that signalled difficulties were entirely consistent with psychiatric models: voices coming from the television and paranoia (2). It may be that this notion of 'split personality' is meaningful because it does give expression to the very powerful feeling, discussed in Chapter 3, that the person has changed in a fundamental way:

> LR: It was the first time I'd experienced anything like that. Alright one minute, and then [1]....

MR: She'd sit there talking to you, this is where it started from and you'd have the television as it is now. She would say 'Liz, they're talking about me, they're coming to get me', and that's where it started building up from there. And then you'd go round and see her: 'Liz the man on the television is after me, they're upstairs' [2] . . . things started coming out.

Some interviewees were very aware and knowledgeable about the psychiatric term that was being employed but still did not actually accord it a great deal of significance. For example, right at the end of this interview with Fred Bryant, I found myself in difficulty introducing the subject of illness. His son, John, had been involved in prostitution a couple of years before. My bringing up of the word 'illness' raises fears about Aids. This accent on the word illness is striking because otherwise Mr Bryant had a distinctly medical view of his son's mental health difficulties. To diffuse any problems, I mention the word 'schizophrenia' (which I usually avoided) and what is noticeable is that Mr Bryant is very familiar with, and even quite knowledgeable about, the term. The reason for him not mentioning it before appears to be that it is simply a term that he accords with little meaning; it is just a name, 'a handle' (1) for which he had little use. He also seemed to question the categorical nature of the diagnosis in defining madness (2):

DJ: Have they talked about John having an illness?
FB: Who?
DJ: People at the hospital . . .
FB: Talked about John having an illness? What do you mean by an illness?
DJ: Well, have they named any illness?
FB: No. I've asked them. Do they think he's got Aids?
DJ: No, an illness like schizophrenia, or . . .
FB: Yeah, they say he's got schizophrenia. I thought you meant he's got Aids, I don't know, that would be possible. But I think they have blood tests there. . . . But if there's anything they should tell me if there's anything wrong with him. . . . But I mean this schizophrenia, I read loads of books, it's just a name in't it? All different psychiatrists have got different opinions about it. What is it? It's just a name, just a handle isn't it [1]? I mean you think about normal behaviour but most murders are committed by people who are supposed to be alright, aren't they? Not by mental patients, so who's . . . who's nuts? [2]

Some interviewees, whilst apparently accepting the psychiatric label, actually seem to have adopted the popular definition of schizophrenia as 'split personality'. The Cook family (it is Arthur's mother and brother, John, talking in the extract below) seem to hold this popular view (1) but they are puzzled and express dissatisfaction with the level of communication (2) and the degree of understanding which professionals have of them (3):

JOHN C: I think the diagnosis is ... er schizophrenia.
MRS C: We got this letter from the social worker with his life story.
JOHN C: That must have been sparse, they don't know much.
MRS C: Well, a history.
JOHN C: They said 'schizophrenia' but there was no explanation of what schizophrenia meant in his individual case. ... I know it's supposed to be split personality [1], a sort of Jekyll and Hyde thing, but what does that mean [2], what are the personalities he has? ... They [professionals] have no comprehension of what it is like to be in a family with someone with mental illness [3].

Vicky Reece also sees schizophrenia as meaning 'split personality' (1), but is equally unsure what that means in her sister's case (2). She has done her own reading (3) and has understood that there is some connection with hereditary (4). This does not, she feels, make that much sense (5). She has also picked up something about childhood deprivation, but that makes little sense to her either (6). Ideas about the causes of mental illness are explored in Chapter 5.

DJ: Did they talk about what sort of illness that Eric [Vicky's brother] or your sister may have?
VR: No, they just said Eric might be schizophrenic and Selena was just depression....
DJ: What about with Eric, what did schizophrenia mean to you?
VR: Split personality [1].
DJ: Does that seem to make sense?
VR: Erm.... No, not really [2] but when I read up about it [3], a lot of people inherit it [4], but er ... I've never seen my mum and dad have a split personality, everyone gets annoyed sometimes [5]... and I didn't see what caused him to go to that, 'cos he was very spoilt [6], got away with murder. And he was a love child.

But with Selena, being the youngest and twins they probably felt a bit left out.

Diane Mason, despite being a qualified nurse working in the health service, also seemed to have the popular understanding of schizophrenia:

> DJ: Being medically qualified, what does schizophrenia mean to you?
>
> DM: Well, split personality, I mean that would be my one- or two-word [definition], split personality...

This lack of use of, or scepticism towards, the diagnostic categories of course reflects the real difficulties that exist, particularly in psychiatry, about diagnosis (Boyle 1990; Mishler 1981; Pilgrim and Rogers 1993). It could also be argued, however, that this scepticism might be a reflection of the poor relationships that seem often to exist between the families and professionals (Creer 1975; Hatfield 1984). The next section will examine this relationship a little closer and suggest that there are disputes over the control of knowledge which contribute to the often poor relationships between families and professionals.

4.2 The Relationship with Professionals: Poor Communication and the Control of Knowledge

The apparent reluctance of medical professionals to use psychiatric diagnoses has been noted for some time (Field 1976). This stands in contrast to consistent findings of physicians' often overzealous use of diagnostic categories (Scheff 1966), although there are other examples of lay demands for diagnosis (Williams and Popay 1994, for example). Mary Galton, a woman in her late twenties, is a good example of someone who gets little information from professionals. The word 'schizophrenic' has been mentioned (1), which she seems to associate with a popular understanding: 'means a person that changes' (2).

> DJ: Did anyone ever give a name to the illness?
>
> MG: Um...not really, they said, I think schizophrenic [1]?
>
> DJ: Mmm, what did that mean to you?
>
> MG: That means a person that changes just like that [2], but I mean to me, I don't think that they can function in society, as a person, really.

Her knowledge of the meaning of 'schizophrenic' might be termed the popular one (split personality: 'a person that changes just like that'). A little later, in response to a specific question about her relationship with professionals, Mary states that she obtains very little information from them. She also seems very aware of there being a power differential operating in her relationship with professionals (1). Not only is there a paucity of information, but she feels that she is not valued by them (4). Mary Galton suggests that there are no grounds for constructive communication between herself and professionals. Mary feels that she does not use the right terminology, does not know the right questions to ask (2). She also expresses clear scepticism about the efficacy of the treatment that is offered to her sister (an issue that will be returned to in the next section) (3):

DJ: How did they [professionals] respond to you, how did they treat you?

MG: Well when I did ask questions they just sort of looked at me as if to say: Who the hell am I, to be asking these questions? [1] They tried to be helpful by fobbing me off. That was their way of being helpful. I didn't know the terminology, I don't know it up to this day; you know, what to ask, what not to ask [2]. I can only ask what I see and they wasn't very helpful. 'Come back and speak to the doctor', 'When would the doctor be available?' well, such and such, you get there and the doctor's not available. It just seems to be drugs, drugs, drugs all the time [3].

DJ: Do you think they were interested in what you had to say . . . as someone who knows Rachael?

MG: No, they didn't seem to be. . . . No they didn't seem to be interested [4].

Mary Galton was a black, working-class, single mother. It might be supposed that there are issues of class and ethnicity, making communication with professionals difficult (Littlewood and Lipsedge 1989). However, the poor relationships that relatives report having with mental health professionals have been consistently documented for some time now (Creer 1975; Cournoyer and Johnson 1991; Holden and Lewine 1982; Mills 1962; Shepherd, Murray and Muijen 1994; Strong 1997). Other people interviewed, such as the Peters family and Jean Karajac, who had more middle-class backgrounds, were equally dissatisfied with how difficult it was to get information from mental health professionals. They did, however, have access to other sources of information. In these cases it was the NSF (National Schizophrenia Fellowship) and SANE (Schizophrenia: A National Emergency) respectively.

Mrs Peters and her daughter Carol were interviewed together. Carol describes her brother's sudden admittance to psychiatric hospital from his workplace. In trying to find out what had happened, the trauma seemed, certainly with hindsight, to have been exacerbated by professionals who seemed particularly unhelpful. The following extract gives a sense of their bewilderment, horror, and the anger that they feel towards professionals:

CP: ...my sister and I were phoning up trying to find out what happened, and they had all been instructed at the company not to tell me and eventually after about 24 hours I got hold of a personnel lady there who I knew, and I said 'You have got to tell me, something has happened, I know he's not been well but something has happened, I feel it, you've got to tell me'. She said 'Look I'll give you this telephone number and you phone the doctor direct'. And what I couldn't believe was his attitude. He, he just, I got on the phone and I said 'I'm Donald Peters' sister and I'm ringing on behalf of my family to find out about Donald Peters' and he said 'What do you want to find out?' So I said 'Well one, where he is...I gather he came to see you, can you tell me what was wrong?' 'What do you think was wrong?' So I said 'Well I don't know, that's why I'm asking you'. So he said 'Go on, you're a clever girl, you tell me what do you think was wrong?' I couldn't believe...I said 'Look I'm sorry I really don't know, I suppose maybe he might have had a nervous breakdown or something'. He said 'That's it, he's loony'.

MRS P: No, 'He's schizophrenic', at least that's what he said to me.

CP: No he didn't, he said to me 'He's completely and utterly loony'. And I said...he said 'Why don't you think you've been told?' I said 'I really don't know', he said 'Go on tell me'. 'Well I suppose the stigma attached to people that are mentally ill'...I was just flabbergasted sitting on the end of this phone. He said 'Yes I sent him down to [general hospital] yesterday morning and that's where he is, under observation, and the family are not allowed to see him until the observation has been done and they've determined what they will do to Donald'. I couldn't believe it.

The Peters' efforts to get information from professionals seemed to be fruitless. These people were white, they could probably be described as upper middle class, and they were certainly articulate. In their relations with professionals, however, they clearly felt utterly powerless and frustrated. Mrs Peters has now acquired a great deal of knowledge about psychiatric matters (sometimes quoting figures to me on suicide rates, or mentioning innovative schemes that she has heard about, for example). She gets her information from the NSF. Her initial contact with the NSF was purely fortuitous (through a friend of a friend), as was Jean Karajac's contact with SANE, described below. Rogers, Pilgrim and Lacey (1993) drew particular attention to the positive views of services provided by voluntary-sector groups (such as MIND) in their survey of psychiatric service user views. They suggest the more informal and less hierarchical relationships within voluntary organizations may have been valued. To Mrs Peters and Jean Karajac the power equation is quite clear – they get information from the voluntary sector and not from professionals.

Jean Karajac greatly appreciates the information that SANE were willing to give him. To Jean, professionals seemed to actively withhold information (as Strong 1997 also reported families feeling). He felt as though they were 'threatened' by his asking questions. Most of the information he has gathered has come from SANE (2). Not only is there information available through SANE (1), but there is a sense of his being able to relate to others, finding that he is not alone (2). It is important to note that he still values the information even when that information is far from optimistic (3, 4). The psychological utility of a certain amount of pessimism is discussed later in Chapter 8 (pp. 135–53).

> I just phoned up [SANE] and said 'Can you give us some information?' They basically sent loads of literature down, which was very helpful and very supportive [1]. You realize that you're not isolated, you know there are a lot of people going through exactly the same crisis as yourself [2]. And you can talk frankly; they basically said 'Well the medication that she is on is all there is, but it's not perfect' [3]. You know like all the doctors come across saying 'Oh this is the cure, this is it!'.... The whole point that annoys me is the medical profession won't recognize that, won't admit that they haven't got any answers [4].

4.2.1   The Use of Knowledge

Sam Mason, from his experiences of considerable contact with professionals concerning his brother, has become particularly sceptical about how formal diagnoses are used or withheld. Sam draws attention to the machinations of power that might underlie the use of certain diagnoses. Disputes over diagnosis are construed by him as revolving around the provision of resources (1), in that a diagnosis of schizophrenia would entail the health service accepting responsibility. Again there is the strong awareness of a power differential in terms of whose perspective can be accepted. There is no sense of shared understanding being reached with the professionals. He certainly did not feel listened to (2). However humorously he presents some of his frustration in the following extract, there is clearly deep frustration and distress; 'torment' (3) is the word he uses.

SM: ... But you don't feel that the society, that the system will really provide anything. Because I don't think they understand it, to be honest, to be honest I don't think they really understand mental illness, because when I'm talking to some of the psychiatrists, they are mad, really! [laughing]. They really are, they are crazy. Because you'll be telling them, you'll be, you'll be the member of the family and you'll be saying 'This person is doing this and this person is not doing this, they're not thinking in this way', and they'll be saying 'There's nothing wrong, they've just got a slight behavioural problem!' or [laughing] ...

DJ: Why do you think they said that?

SM: Because they are mad! [laughing]. ... No, I don't know how much society really wants to care for these people, and sometimes I think that they say 'Yeh, fob them off to the family, let the family deal with them'. If they do say there is something wrong then they may feel that they have to do something about it and that may cost time and money, or whatever [1]. And the system is not geared for that, the system is not really geared for that, so the professional people do say ... like his doctor said he had 'a slight behavioural problem', and this is after years of going in and out of hospital, after years of that doctor seeing him and giving the diagnosis that he was schizophrenic ... he's going: 'It was a behavioural problem', then he said something like 'He's extrovert' [laughing], this is before the last admission into hospital! So I'm led to the conclusion that they are crazy, they're absolutely crazy! ... But we can be saying for months that something is going to happen [2], you know he's on a knife's edge; something's going to happen. But then he'll be at the doctor and the doctor will say 'Oh, he's alright ... not quite alright but almost alright.' It's sad, it really is, cos I'd say for the family it is a lot of torment [3], you know to see someone of your family in a position with him, him going down.

Sam was a black Londoner and his sister, in an earlier interview, had raised the issue of ethnicity and alluded to her feeling of estrangement from professionals (Littlewood and Lipsedge 1989). Sam saw things slightly differently, which emphasizes how great care must be taken in generalizing about attitudes of 'ethnic groups' (Ahmad 1996). He did not feel that there was a problem with racism in the mental health services, at least in the very multicultural area he lived in. He thought that people's prejudices about mental illness were more prominent. He did, however, observe that he felt that MIND (National Association for Mental Health) who were singled out for positive comment by Rogers, Pilgrim and Lacey (1993), was 'for middle class white people'.

It is important to note that, despite his reservations about professionals and their diagnostic categories, Sam sees the diagnosis of schizophrenia as meaningful in that his understanding of the term accords with his observations of his brother (again Sam makes recourse to the notion of split personality (1)):

DJ: I know you say you don't *know*, but how would you diagnose what has happened to Charlie, do you see him as suffering from an illness?

SM: Oh definitely, definitely, I mean they've said 'schizophrenia' and that would, from what I understand of it, would seem to be the illness. Because he does at times behave rationally, he's still able to survive even when he's not well.

DJ: So what does schizophrenia mean to you?

SM: Well to me, as an ignorant person of mental terms, [it] is some-one who behaves, who has got a split personality [1]. And there is a time when you'll be talking to him and he's totally rational, and there is a time when you'll be talking to him when he'll not be taking on board what you're saying.

4.3 Beliefs about Treatment

It is clear that the people interviewed saw their relatives as suffering from an illness. They did not, however, necessarily construe that illness in formal psychiatric terms. Indeed, relationships between themselves and professionals were viewed quite negatively. Communication certainly appeared poor. An exploration of the relatives' attitudes towards the treatments that were made available provides further evidence of the distinctly weak relationship that they had with psychiatry. Their beliefs about psychiatric treatment are fairly easy to summarize: they are marked by ambivalence (much in keeping with survey work on psychiatric service users, beliefs about treatments – Rogers, Pilgrim and Lacey 1993). There is a clear perception that the main treatment that is offered is drug treatment. Whilst it was usually believed that medication was essential to avoid further deterioration or breakdown, there was scepticism about the efficacy of the medication. No one saw the medication as representing any kind of cure and there was concern about the side-effects.

Similarly, ambivalence about the therapeutic value of psychiatric hospitals was frequently expressed. The local old asylum hospital (Friern), was often singled out as an unpleasant environment, but it was also recognized that it did provide some support for people. Some people wished that there was more exploration of 'talking cures', or that the whole situation of their relatives needed to be addressed in a manner that had not been happening (again rather similar to the service users' views presented by Rogers, Pilgrim and Lacey 1993).

4.3.1 Medication

Molly Quinn is quite typical here of someone who, whilst not overtly hostile to the mental health professionals, is, however, quite sceptical about what power they have to help her sister. Contrast is made with physical medicine (1):

DJ: Have you found that hospital staff and doctors have talked to you about what's going on?

MQ: Well not in great detail, no, not at all in fact . . . only what I've asked.

DJ: Have they been helpful when you've asked?

MQ: Yes they have been, but you see it's, . . . I suppose at any level of mental illness it's really experimenting, not experimenting but trying to stabilize each patient and it's a case of trying out different things, isn't it? So it comes back to the old story, if you've got a broken leg people know exactly what to do, but with mental illness even the doctors sometimes are trying this, try that, sometimes aren't they? [1]

Molly Quinn described with concern some serious side-effects which her sister had suffered from at one point. Nevertheless, when asked whether she thought the medication was helpful:

MQ: ...Without, it...it seems to be the only thing that stabilizes her, I don't know whether she would stabilize without it in time, I don't know. I just don't know. I think that she does need something to keep her fairly normal, because when she refuses to take something she goes completely, er...well withdrawn, out of this world.

Similarly Diane Mason, in this notable exchange (her mother MM is also present), explains that she values the medication because it controls her brother Charlie in a way that enables him to play a part in family life. Diane feels the medication enables him to fulfil a reasonably normal role as father when his estranged children visit. Without medication Charlie is considered too destructive, which worries Diane particularly as she herself has a young child. The significance of these comments about fitting in with family life will become clearer in later chapters. It will be argued that being able to fulfil certain familial roles is an important part of the definition of sanity (see Chapter 7, particularly).

DJ: Do you think the medication is a big help?
DM: It's something he requires...
MM: Calms him down.
DM: All the time, or even I mean it's something he needs at first and if he's on it all the time it should keep him on an even keel, so that he can fit in, you know, like his children were down for Easter, even though he sort of didn't go round, take them out, they were down and I think he felt....
MM: Oh yeah, he was playing cards with them and things like that, don't talk a lot.
DM: The kids look forward, because what are they, 15 now? They sort of came down to see their dad, that helps him a bit. Basically what it is, I mean he's lonely in the flat, ...when he gets a bit aggressive, we can tolerate him for so long but then it is stressful for us to have him all the time if he is going to behave in a way that is not acceptable...I mean that upsets our lives as well, I've got a son, you can't have him swearing 'round him whatever. So we can only tolerate so much – if he's on medication, he's more acceptable, he's more likely to be included in what

we are doing. If he's not on medication then you know unfortunately he's not, he's not acceptable, his behaviour is not acceptable to us.

The Cooks were quite hostile to the professional services, feeling that they had particularly failed to understand their experiences as a black family. They saw them as having let their son down, and their view of medication fits in with this. When I ask about medication, his mother tells me, 'Oh yes, the injections and the manner they have been given have not been satisfying at all, they just put him to sleep at night.' The father then asks me if I had heard a story that had recently been publicized about a black man in a secure hospital being killed by being given too large an injection. It is pointed out, with significance, that Arthur too has been forced to accept injections. Arthur's younger brother John expressed his opinion on medication when I asked the family whether they saw Arthur as ever getting better, becoming the person he had been. 'No', John replied, 'for two reasons; firstly, the length of time it's been now and, secondly, the amount of drugs he had will have a long-term effect.'

Jean Karajac describes an awareness of the contradictory benefits of the medication that his sister receives. It is, again, interesting to note that his information comes not from professionals but from SANE:

DJ: Do you see the medication as being a big help?

JK: Well, if it weren't for SANE I know, basically the medication – all it is is a hyped-up tranquillizer. All it does is get rid of the voices, but on the other hand it removes the exhilaration – where she feels special for hearing voices and so on. Which is understandable, it's the only excitement in her life if you like. And then it brings the real depression forward into reality...the depression that is always with her but if you like is pushed below by other things going on in her life, in her mind.

To an extent, of course, the observations about medication might be said to merely reflect the reality of this group's circumstances. These were relatives of a group who are seen as having long-term difficulties, who by definition have not been 'cured' or very significantly helped. Nevertheless, the ambivalence is noteworthy. Even amongst those who saw medication as being a great help, concern was still often expressed about the side-effects of the drugs. This ambivalence is carried forward into their views about hospitals.

4.3.2   Views about Hospital

Jean Karajac's sister had just been admitted to an acute psychiatric ward in a general hospital. He was clearly sceptical about the value of hospital care (here he is referring to an acute ward in a general hospital) as being anything other than a short-term measure that would achieve little:

> JK: Already it looks like she'll sit there for 28 days, and she's complaining herself. I went to see her last night, she's finally calmed down, she's been in for 5 days, she's on medication. OK she wanders off into the delusions and the voices intermittently... between that she'll say 'What's the point of me being here? All I do is sit here – they don't make me do anything.' And you understand the fact that they are short-staffed and so on, but what is the point of going into hospital? It's going to be the same old cycle.

Fred Bryant referred to the old asylum hospital as appearing 'like something out of a horror movie' when he first saw it. He very forcefully expressed his antipathy towards the hospital, focusing particularly on the apparent lack of contact that his son has with staff. Nevertheless, he does feel great conflict in that he also acknowledged that he has been grateful to be able to turn to the hospital as a place where he can get some refuge by their taking his son.

One quite common criticism of the hospital was that patients were just allowed to come and go as they pleased, the implication being that one thing the hospital could provide was custodial care. Typical were Mr and Mrs Regan, who told several stories about how Mrs Regan's sister had wandered off the ward with few clothes, even in very cold weather. Or she had gone home and simply neglected herself. They very clearly wanted the hospital to take care, and custody, of Cathy. The dilemmas presented by wishing for new forms of asylum are discussed from a variety of perspectives in Carrier and Tomlinson (1996).

4.4   Summary: the Relationship with Psychiatry

In summary, it does not seem as though psychiatry and the allied professions are directly forcing a medicalized view onto the families (Mishler 1981). In fact, what emerges is a curious story in which the majority of relatives interviewed felt that professionals were very reluctant to share psychiatric information – or any other kind of information – with them. Where people did seem to have considerable psychiatric knowledge, they had usually obtained it elsewhere: from their own reading, from friends or voluntary groups such as the NSF or SANE. The picture that emerges is of the relatives asking, even begging, for information which professionals, from the point of view of these interviewees, seem to withhold.

Sam Mason (p. 63) seems clearly to perceive that the illness model not only provides meaning to him, but it provides instrumental meaning: if professionals recognize the medical nature of his brother's difficulties then they have to shoulder more of the responsibility. Thus one explanation of the antipathy between families and the professionals they have contact with is suggested here by Sam Mason's insight into the power struggle involved in the construction of his brother's difficulties. Power and knowledge are joined together in the construction of these people's mental health problems. Conflict thus emerges in disputes over the communication and sharing of information.

The families, reporting of a paltry level of information coming from psychiatrists and other professionals does not suggest that these interviewees are having a psychiatric model imposed upon them. These relatives do not seem to be simply adopting the 'professional' models with which they are being presented. What I want to argue is that this suggests that what we think of as 'psychiatric models' of mental illness have not been created solely by those professional groups. Instead they have the same common roots in our culture as the 'lay beliefs' of these relatives. To understand attitudes towards people with mental health problems we need to look beyond the models provided by professionals. As discussed in Chapter 1, there is some historical support for this view, in that families seemed to be involved in identifying mental illnesses during the nineteenth century when the asylums were being built. Nancy Tomes (1994: 92), writing on the creation of a North American asylum in the nineteenth century, observed that 'regardless of their varying levels of sophistication, the patrons [families] all employed the same basic language of disease: Individuals were spoken of as "sick" or "unwell"'. Tomes argues that the asylums were constructed through the active co-operation of medical staff and the families who were unable to cope. It would seem from examination of my interviews with families that, at the turn of the twentieth century, they also see their relatives' difficulties in straightforward terms of illness. Whilst 'co-operation' is not a word that they would generally use about their relationships with mental health professionals, it must be recognized that the relatives are being very *active* in their use of the concepts of illness. The next chapter will explore in more detail the ideas that family members had about the causes of mental illness. What emerges is how active people are in their search for meaningful ideas that will help them understand their relatives' difficulties. In addition, the pathways that people follow in pursuing those meanings are negotiated through the wider webs of feelings and relationships in which people are involved.

5

The Moral Construction of Diagnosis: 'Sickness made for anyone'

The previous chapters have argued that families are likely to feel as though they had lost the relative they knew and were therefore experiencing a complex grief. It has already been observed that families seemed to make recourse, with little hesitation, to a medical understanding of what had happened. The evidence of the previous chapter suggests that it might be wrong to suppose that the families were simply internalizing the model of illness from professionals. This chapter will explore the ideas that families had about what might have caused their relatives' difficulties. These relatives generally held eclectic and often complex views. This finding that individuals could make use of different theories is in keeping with Furnham and Bower's (1992) work on lay beliefs about mental illness and more general work on Western lay beliefs (Fitzpatrick 1989). This chapter is written with the aim of looking beneath that eclecticism in order to chart the forces that are shaping those ideas. Those forces, it will be argued, reveal a more complicated picture than that suggested by the idea that psychiatric diagnoses arise simply from the medicalization of Western culture.

All of the interviewed families were concerned with finding reasons for their relatives' suffering in ways that were meaningful to them. At times there is a sense of there being a quite desperate scrabble for meaning, with no stone being left unturned in the search for the right theory. Perelberg (1983a, 1983b), in her study of families and mental illness, referred to families being involved in a 'search for meaning'. However, analysis of what underlies this search suggests that it is better seen as *a struggle* for meaning. The theories are all shaped by a complex array of often powerful emotions. Feelings of anger, guilt and shame can be traced within the theories that people held. The theories also carry complex moral implications. In searching out theories of cause,

71

there is a concern with blame (as in what has happened in the past) and responsibility (as in what should happen now and in the future).

I would argue that the scrabbling for ideas and theories reflects a need that people have to find meaning, to place themselves and their experiences within meaningful frameworks (Mishler 1981). Lévi-Strauss (1969) wrote of the exemplary roles of the psychoanalyst of modern Western society and the shaman of South American cultures in putting people's experiences into discourse. He describes the efficacy of the cure of the shaman of the South American Indian:

> The cure would consist, therefore, in making explicit a situation originally existing on the emotional level and in rendering acceptable to the mind pains which the body refuses to tolerate. That the mythology of the shaman does not correspond to an objective reality does not matter... What she [the 'patient'] does not accept are the incoherent and arbitrary pains, which are an alien element in her system but which the shaman, calling upon myth, will re-integrate within a whole where everything is meaningful.   (Lévi-Strauss 1968: 197)

Perhaps this parallels these interviewees' need for knowledge very well. In gathering terms, facts and figures about mental illness, or elaborating theories and scenarios, they are defending themselves from what are otherwise 'incoherent and arbitrary pains' (Lévi-Strauss 1968: 197). This is an important theme, which will be explored in greater detail in the following chapters.

Within the theories held by the relatives interviewed, there was often an immanent concern with moral responsibility. It becomes clear that people are very aware that theories of mental illness carry moral implications. The ill person was rarely seen as being responsible for their condition, but other people would often be accused. Greenberg, Kim and Greenley (1997) found that feelings of subjective burden were lower amongst siblings of people with severe mental illness when they saw the cause of the illness as lying outside the sufferer's control. Similarly, Robinson (1996) found that families who avoided blaming people are able to function better than those who do blame, and suggests this may be connected to people's 'attributional style' – that is, non-blaming attributions might reflect a generally more optimistic outlook. It will be argued here, through a detailed examination of what people had to say about the causes of illness, that the ideas people had were deeply embedded within their own, often unacknowledged, feelings of aggression, guilt and shame. The discussion in Chapter 3 stressed how anger was likely to be a very natural part of people's responses to mental illness. In this chapter we will begin to see how other emotions, such as guilt and shame, are also commonly present. It will be argued here that it is not that people's *ideas* about mental illness cause 'ugly' feelings. Those feelings are already there, provoked by the distressing things that people are faced with. The theories about cause are an aspect of the families' struggle for meaning, for finding a safe conduit for some of those feelings. The struggle the relatives are involved in is in trying to put those painful feelings into systems of discourse where they can be comprehensible. What is also clear is that people were using their own resources of knowledge and experience to build up their own explanatory models. The interviews were caried out in an area that had become notorious for poor relationships between police and local youth (particularly from ethnic minorities). This local experience made its appearance in the ideas a number of the families (mainly, but not exclusively, Afro-Caribbean families) had about police ill treatment contributing to, or triggering, illness.

What emerges in this chapter is the manner in which these so-called lay beliefs are in themselves inseparable from Foucault's power and knowledge couple (Foucault 1977). This suggests that ideas about mental illness are not emerging solely from the scientific discourses, and power machinations, of professional elites but are immanent to much wider cultural needs. This supports Barham's (1992: 140) view that the role that psychiatrists have played in the medicalization and confinement of insanity has not been as 'overlords of independent fiefdoms', but rather as 'lieutenants' of more powerful social processes. Tomes (1994: 12), also, concludes of the American asylum that it 'was not the sole creation of doctors or lay reformers, ... but an institution sanctioned by the whole society to meet certain commonly perceived needs'.

Section 1 of this chapter will argue that people's awareness of moral responsibility could be detected in their thoughts about the causes of their relative's difficulties. These theories seemed to form safe conduits for their feelings of anger, and provided some protection from feelings of guilt. Section 2 will discuss some of the limitations of this latter strategy, as it becomes clear that some relatives do feel that they are blamed by others (and perhaps they do blame themselves). These experiences of blame and guilt are very shameful and difficult to discuss. Discussion of the significance of shame will be developed fully in the next chapter, but its influence will be briefly considered in Section 3, in relation to people's seeming reluctance to discuss theories of genetic influences. Feelings about genetics and mental illness are clearly sensitive since they may present parents with the idea that they have 'given' mental illness to their children, and may leave other family members with the feeling that they also share this genetic trait. Whilst genetic theories become more prevalent, these are important issues in themselves. The argument, taken further in the next chapter, is that feelings about genetics reveal something about the (perhaps unconscious) identifications that relatives may have with one another. Section 4 will discuss the prominence of theories about broken hearts and sexual/romantic relationships. These ideas were a notable departure from official psychiatric explanations. This not only emphasizes how psychiatric discourses and the relatives' discourses were not entirely continuous, but also leads to consideration of the importance attributed to sexuality in the definition of normality. It is important to note how *actively* the relatives are themselves defining the boundaries between sanity and 'madness'. The priority given to sexuality, which emerges alongside the influence of guilt, shame and ager within theories of cause, points to the importance of the analysis of the emotional nature of the interviewees, perceptions of, and their attachments to, their relatives.

The findings discussed here should be noted particularly by professionals working with families. It will be argued that the complexity of people's explanations sometimes only really emerged when people were given space to communicate (Mathieson 1999), and sometimes the important feelings of shame often revealed themselves only during the gaps, or in the seeming failures of dialogue in the interview itself.

5.1 Moral Implications: Feelings of Guilt and Blame

It has already been suggested in Chapter 3 that the medical model provided a safe target for the feelings of anger that are likely to be a natural response amongst relatives (Kinsella, Anderson and Anderson 1996). Angermeyer and Matschinger (1996) surveyed members of Austrian and German associations for relatives of people with schizophrenia diagnoses and found they were more likely than people from the general population to believe in the biomedical model of mental illness. They suggest this may partly be a function of their need to assuage feelings of guilt. Mr Doors is perhaps a good example of someone who has some emotional investment in the organic model that might partly be explained by his feelings of guilt. His investment is perhaps signalled by his spontaneous use of a psychiatric diagnosis which, as discussed in Chapter 3, was relatively unusual. Mr Doors's daughter's biological mother had died when April was three, and he subsequently married a woman who treated her badly. Mr Doors ruminated a good deal on whether this ill treatment lay at the root of his daughter's difficulties, which perhaps in part explains why he was particularly anxious for information. It is a desire for information seemingly not satisfied by staff:

DJ: At these various points were they [psychiatric hospital staff] discussing with you what they thought was going on?

JD: Oh no, no!...I don't know if there was a change in the political climate as it were, I think in the past two, three years people actually telling me what they thought was wrong; before that either they didn't tell me or they wouldn't commit themselves. I said 'Well, is she manic-depressive?'...either they didn't want to tell me or they didn't know...when I pushed the point they said 'Well mental medicine isn't like physical, it isn't straightforward, it isn't black and white'....It's all very evasive. No one was even able to tell me whether the treatment that April had from her stepmother – of course I should never have allowed it to take place in the first place really – ...um, whether that affected her, or would it be inborn? And no one could categorically say 'yes' or 'no'. Some people said 'Well, the general opinion is that it wouldn't'.

To Mr Doors the medical model is perhaps a source of some comfort as it suggests that his daughter's difficulties are not due to her stepmother's maltreatment (and his non-intervention). This pattern whereby the model that supposes a disease with organic roots is contrasted with a model that blames the family environment was not uncommon. In many cases the situation is more complicated than this, however. Another dimension of 'moral responsibility' can be seen to emerge in the following interview with Jean Karajac, as we begin to sense some of the complicated feelings he has that shape the accusation (Perelberg 1983a) of blame that he makes.

In supposing that he and his sister's upbringing was odd, and that his sister's difficulties might be caused by that upbringing, he reveals some feelings about his own childhood. The family was isolated (2), perhaps he and his siblings were overprotected (3) and spoilt (4). Jean wonders if the reason for him not becoming ill was his own strength (5). However, the knowledge that he acquired about the medical model of schizophrenia (from friends) has now 'tempered' this view (1). Hereditary is also vaguely considered (6) – the ambivalent feelings about genetic links are discussed in Section 3 of this chapter:

DJ: What do you think happened now...have you any thoughts about why, what caused it?

JK: Er, I really don't know. It's been tempered [1] by what I know, from my friends, that schizophrenia is a medical disease, they discovered that quite recently. I always [thought] about the family...we were a very close-knit family, very isolated [2], all our relatives actually live abroad. My father wasn't a very greg-arious person, he had a few choice, close friends, always pro-tected us maybe too much [3], my mother definitely spoils us too much [4]. She always believed her job was to look after us and do everything for us and I spent many a time in my adolescence sort of fighting that, trying to do my own thing! And I had the strength to do that [5], my sister never did. I'd say I had the confidence of a great circle of friends and my sister always found it very dif-ficult to make friends, she was always very shy. I'd say I was shy when I was younger but I was fortunate in a lot of ways in having such good contacts. I always had my own networks, she never did and that made it very difficult for her, coupled with the fact that me and my brother were academically successful in school and she wasn't. Which left her with a crisis of confidence, what was she going to be good at? Where is her niche in society? And I don't think she saw one, and all those pressures were pulled down on her, plus the fact on my dad's side I know there is schizophrenia running through his side of the family [6]...I don't know whether that can lead to it in any way.

Mr and Mrs Snellman also saw hereditary factors being involved in their cousin's illness, but also felt that his upbringing might be involved as well. His mother died when he was young and he was brought up between his father and grandmother. The behaviour of Erik's grandmother and father was seen as being part of the problem. This hypothesis was raised with considerable feeling (they did not like his grandmother), revealing clearly a moral dimension. Later in the interview it becomes apparent that the placing of responsibility else-where, in that he 'had it rough from all sides' (1), forms part of a rea-soning that allows the person or self of the sufferer to remain intact. He is still lovable and innocent 'underneath it all' (2), the blame lies elsewhere:

MRS S: Yes, this was a poor young man who had it rough from all sides [1], and basically he was a lovable, loving child and everything has gone wrong and underneath it all there is still a loveable person [2]. but you can hardly ever get to it, and you certainly can't get close. I mean when I said once, 'Since we lost our daughter, we are frightened of the future, of getting old like everyone else...'...Our son lives in Poole his wife is very nice, but it's all very different, and he sort of hugged me and said 'Oh Peggy I'll always look after you', you know the heart is there, but the illness doesn't give him a chance...

Fred Bryant, being separated from his son's mother, could perhaps also afford to lay blame at her door (1). At the same time he wonders about drug abuse (2), and notes that his son was different earlier, as a teenager (3):

DJ: What do you think caused the illness?
FB: Well it may be something from his mother [1], but she had two other children and they're perfectly alright...er it could have been, if stuff was put in his drink it could have been a real blummin' overdose of acid [2] which might have done something. He's certainly, since then, not been right at all. Before that he wasn't right, in that he wasn't mixing with people, he wasn't a teenager as such [3], he was just keeping entirely on his own.

Later on in the interview the idea that John may have received a blow to the head is aired (1). Again the expression of anger (in this case directed against the police) is clear:

...I don't know what happened that night he's supposed to have smashed up three police cars, I don't know if he was banged about the head [1], I really literally do not know....All I know is that from that night when that incident took place John has not been, he's not been right. Where before he was strange, after that night he was gone....

It is important to note how different theories could be held by the same person (Young 1981). The fact that Mr Bryant (like many other interviewees) could hold these different theories is an important point about this style of interviewing families. A very different impression might have been reached had people been straightforwardly asked what they believed was the cause and had they not been given space to expand on their thinking (Mathieson 1999).

Mr Ajani was another father who wondered if ill treatment at the hands of authorities had made his son ill. To Mr Ajani, the fact that his son was black was a factor leading to his being picked on by the police. Whilst Mr Ajani's observations may be legitimate (Fernando 1991; Littlewood and Lipsedge 1989), it is clear that some of his own feelings and experiences as a black man in Britain are being brought in here:

DJ: What do you think caused the problems in the first place?

MR A: I'm not a psychiatrist, nor a doctor. What I can say is that they did something to him, kick his head because he had a nose bleed.... They could have done something to him, I'm not very sure how it could have been done, I'm not an expert, but if certain wicked people want to do certain things as I just told you – the police were coming here looking for him because they promised him. A lot of things are wrong in this country....

DJ: Do you think that it was as a black person that he was treated particularly badly?

MR A: Yes I'm sure it was. I'm not a racist – but I know – they think every black man is a thief and if you are a black man you are bad. Forgetting that you take people as you find them, it's just... I've been in this country, next June it will be 20 years, I got no single criminal record. But certain parts of the authorities, especially the police, I hated them – especially this area they are no good.

Diane Mason also expressed anger about the racist environment that impacted on her brother, although she took a different view of its operation. She wondered if her observation of the over-representation of young black men on psychiatric wards (this is, of course, an accurate observation – King et al. 1994) was due to the fact that their difficulties were not picked up early enough. Perhaps their behaviour was too easily dismissed as being due to 'cultural differences'. Both Diane and her mother adopted theories that implied social causes of illness. The social factors that were put forward were to do with relationship difficulties (with the mother of his children), unemployment and the subsequent poverty and denial of a traditional masculine role. These very notable latter points about the assumed significance of family roles and relationships are discussed at some length in Chapter 7.

Although a number of social factors were put forward by the Masons, they do not suggest that the family might be to blame. This may not be at all surprising, but does emphasize how diagnoses are moral enterprises. Particularly notable was the fact that the Masons did not discuss the hereditary theory. Mrs Mason regularly attended a relatives' group, where they had talks about schizophrenia and mental illness. Her daughter was a nurse (general medical). It was difficult to believe that they had not come across the theory. I spent some considerable time with Mrs Mason in the following months and there was still no mention of a theory of hereditary cause. This raises what I have come to believe to be an important theme: the influence of shame. In that silence, in the omission of the mention of the hereditary hypothesis, there is evidence of the effect of shame in shaping ideas and experiences.

5.2 Ashamed of Blame

Elly Blacksmith is someone whose ideas about cause, and her responses to my questioning about stigma, suggest feelings of shame. She, like other interviewees, mentions several possible causes of her son's difficulties. She thinks it possible that it was to do with smoking cannabis, his religious ideas (of Rastafarianism), and the stress of studying. When asked what the doctors had told her, she takes care to say that her son's difficulties are not seen as to do with the brain (which is 'perfect'), they are to do with 'the mind'. When asked about stigma (in the extract below) however, it becomes clear that despite seeing her son's difficulties as being of the realm of mind, Mrs Blacksmith is adamant that her son's difficulties are those of illness. Perhaps the vehemence of her response to the questioning about feelings of stigma actually suggests that she does experience a certain amount of stigma or blame (1). Perhaps the notion of illness or sickness (being used here to highlight the morally neutral condition of her son) is one that offers some protection from this stigma ('nobody don't go out and buy sickness, sickness made for anyone') (2). The full significance of stigma and shame is returned to in Chapter 6.

DJ: Sometimes other family members often feel that other people look down on them because there is mental illness...?

EB: Well nobody looked down on me 'cos you, they doesn't, you know, nobody looks.... I don't care if anybody want to. I don't care, you know, you've got to hold your head up high. I don't care what nobody says [1], nobody don't go out and buy sickness, sickness made for anyone [2]. So I don't care, my family they love him, all my family love him, they do anything for him, you know if I'm not around they go to him, if I was to go away on holiday... no not with my family because we're such a close-knit family....

Jean Karajac and Molly Quinn (siblings to Janice Karajac and Christine Connor respectively) both talked about how their parents had blamed themselves. Molly Quinn's parents had separated and Molly had initially blamed this disruption for her sister's illness. Her mother's subsequent contact with the NSF had provided a different explanation. There she had met 'couples that have had very happy marriages and very happy family units and their children have still suffered the illness'. This explanation was more palatable to Molly.

Jean Karajac understands that his mother's current high level of involvement with his sister is a function of her feeling of guilt:

My mum is... she reacts so, she feels responsible, without a doubt, I think my father did as well, that's what ended up killing him [he died of a heart attack a few years earlier]. That it's their fault, they still do feel that, they come from, say, an old-fashioned view of mental illness. However much you tell them 'Look don't put it all on yourself', she does. That's why she always visits the hospital every day, she always cooks for my sister every day, she doesn't understand why she doesn't react positively to that, and sometimes negatively, she doesn't realize that sometimes she is actually crowding my sister too much, you know.

Both of these siblings had come across information which persuaded them that the 'dysfunctional family' model of cause was incorrect. It is interesting to observe that nobody interviewed volunteered themselves as being the cause of their relatives' difficulties (the rare exception to this might be Mrs Land, who is discussed on p. 141). In fact I interviewed Jean Karajac's mother, on her own, and despite a great deal of rumination on what had happened to her daughter (pp. 89–90, this chapter, for example) and some blame being apportioned to her late husband, at no point was there any suggestion that she felt guilty in the way that Jean tells me she does. I now wonder whether the admission of having feelings of guilt, which her son talked about, would have evoked such feelings of shame that they could not be easily expressed.

Upon reflection, I think that an interview I carried out with Mrs Murray does provide some support for this notion. This was one of the more difficult interviews to complete (referred to earlier in the section on those who refused to be recorded – Chapter 2, p. 35 and Appendix A). It took several visits to arrange; several times I appeared at the pre-arranged time only to be told that it would not be convenient as she was too busy just then. When I did manage to sit down and speak with Mrs Murray, she refused to be recorded and was quite hostile and suspicious. During the course of the interview, when I asked her whether any particular name of an illness had been mentioned, I was told that she had been informed that her daughter had 'manic depressive illness'. The atmosphere became more contentious when I tried to explore what that meant to her, or whether anyone explained what 'manic depressive illness' might mean. Mrs Murray seemed to feel very uncomfortable. She told me that the doctor at the time said that her daughter's difficulties were caused by the stress of her and her husband's marriage break-up. When I tried to explore how she felt about this accusation, she became very angry, exclaiming 'I don't want to go into my personal details with you!' Assuming that she felt very angry about the injustice of this accusation, I tried to calm things down by pointing out that many people saw this sort of mental illness as just like any other illness, with a physical cause. Mrs Murray told me very firmly that she felt the family background *was* indeed responsible but that she herself did not feel blame as it was her husband who had left *her*. Jane was the eldest and had had the most attention from them both, so she had been most affected by his departure. Her husband's new wife had then not wanted to have anything to do with the children, the explanation continued. I do not think it would be taking too many liberties with interpretation to suggest that Mrs Murray actually felt (however unjustifiably) acutely responsible for her daughter's illness, hence her initial ambivalence about the interview and aggressive response to some of my questioning which was probing about what she thought had caused her daughter's difficulties.

Mr Reece was another parent who seemed to feel rather persecuted by my line of questioning on this matter. It is hard to say whether Mr Reece was harbouring explicit feelings of guilt about causing his son, Eric, to become ill, but he had at one time taken an injunction out against him to prevent him returning to the house because of his violence. In this extract from the interview, Mr Reece has very tentatively proffered an idea that his son's difficulties might have been caused by smoking cannabis (he spoke to a young woman on a psychiatric ward who had told him that is what had caused her difficulties). When I try and pin him down to it he becomes quite defensive about not being able to control what children do, and angry about exploitative drug pushers (1):

DJ: But you think maybe that was it, he was smoking?

MR: Well you can't tell. I just can't tell. 'Cos you asking him, he say 'No'. So how would I know? I never seen him. But this is what I'm saying, from the time your son or the daughter close that door, you is in here. They gone out, gone down that stairs, go up the road, you don't know what they doing. You'll be lucky someone passed them that knows you come in and say 'Oh I see your girl talking to a boy, or I see your boy talking to a girl, they was smoking' or 'They was this', you will be lucky. Just can't tell. But lots of these young people, that is what got them like that. Drugs and smokes and all things like that. Killing themselves. People is making money whilst they is killing themselves [1].

I then (a little insensitively) pursue the matter of what he really believes about cause. As I do so the conversation becomes shorter and shorter:

DJ: Have any doctors since then, or have the [Voluntary Care agency] people, talked about what might have happened?

MR: No . . . I wish someone would tell me. . . . Have you ever been in touch with Eric?

DJ: No, no.

MR: Well I think as a matter of fact he's the one you should really get in touch with, try to find out what caused his illness or anything. Because most probably where he don't tell me, he might tell you. Who knows? And then have you ever been seen by [Voluntary Care Agency] people or anything like that?

DJ: No, no . . .

MR: So who are you only seeing about Eric?

DJ: Just the families of people, to see how they see things.

MR: Yeah but how do you get to know about Eric?

DJ: Oh from the hospital, from the records.

MR: The hospital don't tell you nothing?

DJ: No, I just get the addresses, you see.

MR: Yeah well them is the people to ask, what can we tell you? Because they knows more than me really.

DJ: Yes, but I'm just wondering whether they talk to you, that's . . .

MR: No. No.

DJ: No?

MR: All they say to us, I know once we went down there: 'He's mentally disturbed'.

DJ: Yeah...

MR: What was this mentally disturbed I don't know.

DJ: It seems they haven't told you much at all, they haven't discussed things with you.

MR: ...Well people come around saying they want to find out this and they want to find out that, it's not a lot I can say to them really.

I sense that there is not only a feeling of shame about what had happened; that perhaps he does feel responsible, but that he assumes that my line of questioning suggests that I think he ought to understand why his son had become ill. The one explanation that he has been offered (smoking cannabis) by a patient on the ward is taken up, although with some scepticism since he noted that his son even finds tobacco smoke offensive. It seems as though professionals have not provided alternatives, which he experiences as persecutory. It is worth noting that here I am being bracketed with professionals, since he finds my line of questioning rather harassing.

The interview with Mrs Lord was also a difficult interview. It was not possible to record the interview since she was initially so suspicious (perhaps particularly of a white person), and believed that her son had been treated badly by the system. She was very sceptical about the psychiatric system. She had heard that her son's difficulties 'could be hereditary', but this made no sense since she did not 'have anything like it in my family or his father don't...so how come?' Later, perhaps after I had won a bit of trust, Mrs Lord reveals that she thinks that her son has been a victim of, if not racism, then at least cultural misunderstanding (see Littlewood and Lipsedge 1989 for examples of such misunderstandings). I am told that 'people who come to this country are different – maybe they like to sing to themselves and people say that they are mad and they are not...I don't know, maybe things that they give him make him worse, make him like that, the place they put him maybe, I don't know...maybe they do their best'. Her initial reluctance in being interviewed seems to reflect her feelings towards professionals and the way that she imagines they look at her.

Mrs Teague was also initially suspicious of my presence and refused to be recorded. She seemed unsure and confused about whether she saw her son as suffering from an illness. At one point she thought his mental state was associated with 'bad company...and smoking the weed'. Her husband used to smoke a bit, which was OK, but Simon would smoke all day. When I asked if she thought the illness had led Simon to smoke like that, she told me that she thought 'No, it wasn't illness, it was the company' that Simon got into. I wondered if anyone had talked to her about what had been happening, what was wrong with Simon? Her response was unequivocal: 'No! No one ever talked to me about what's wrong, just ask me to take him.' Professionals seemed to have offered her no alternatives. She is left with the idea that her son has simply turned out bad. I cannot help feeling that it is likely that, as his mother, she has been left with the feeling that she is somehow responsible. This would be very painful and may well explain why she had, for the time being, cut off contact with him.

The difficulty that interviewees experienced in coming to terms with their own feelings, and how this impacts on the sort of relationships they have, will be explored in Chapter 8. These last few examples seem to point to the silencing effect of feelings of shame. Those feelings of being blamed and perhaps ashamed seem to be effectively keeping people out of dialogue with other people, where more constructive and palatable understandings might emerge.

5.3   Shame and Genetics

In order to explore the influence of shame in constructing people's thoughts and views further, it is worth spending some more time looking at the interviews with Jacob Doors. This was a particularly 'open' interviewee, who seemed to use the interviews to think about his relationship to his daughter. It has already been suggested, earlier in this chapter, that Jacob Doors seemed to draw comfort from a biological understanding of his daughter's difficulties. Perhaps this freed him from some feelings of responsibility and guilt about her upbringing (as Angermeyer and Matschinger 1996 suggest). Jacob also talked about his first wife (his daughter's mother) showing psychotic symptoms before her death. When talking to me he seemed to make no link between his late wife's difficulties and those of his daughter. I was curious about this silence, so I wondered what this link between the behaviour of his late wife and daughter had meant to him. There is something about the hesitant and stumbling response which seems to betray a sense of fear and shame about there being a connection, perhaps a genetic link (1):

DJ: But I wonder how you felt when you realized that similar things were happening to April that happened to her mother?

JD: Er...?

DJ: It must affect the way you look at it?

JD: ...I don't think I ever consciously faced the fact as a matter of fact, until you raised the point. I don't think I'd ever consciously raised the fact – I'd thought of it, put it down, and yes obviously borne it in mind, but I didn't actually sit down and... something I didn't want to face, didn't like to face that somebody was genetically condemned to something [1]. I mean, yes... obviously I've thought of that at times. I was just hoping that it would get better in April's case. Now admitted it's lasted a long time so perhaps I shouldn't think that, but when you see someone acting in a bizarre fashion in that split second in time you don't actually get the whole picture. And er... it has... yes I do think about it. It's not, I don't deliberate upon it. I tend to, for instance I think of my son and he's OK, he's very calm, though you could see tiny little things, you don't want to start looking for anything wrong. He is very defensive at times and quite easily upset, although he puts a barrier over it, he's a fireman, and quite a good one at that so he is obviously someone who can handle things. I'm pleased it didn't come out in him. I wonder if he had children if it would come out again or if it watered down – however genetics work. Yes, it was disturbing yes, it was disturbing, but I didn't actually make a point of, um, thinking about the connection over much...

For parents like Mr Doors the anxiety about genetics may well be to do with the fear that they have passed something on. An interview with a sibling also revealed considerable anxiety about genetic links. Mary Galton, when actually asked about her ideas about what had caused her sister's difficulties, responds by suggesting that it was her sister's break-up with her boyfriend (see the next section, 'Madness and a Broken Heart', this chapter, for more on the significance of romantic relationships). Later in the interview, however, Mary herself tentatively mentions that she has been involved in a study looking at genetic links in her family. This is a subject to which she switches out of the blue (1). It seems to be something that she is fearful about. Perhaps it is only after some trust has been won during the interview that she is prepared to share that fear and maybe to seek advice or perhaps reassurance. Obviously I feel rather uncomfortable, wondering what reassurance

I should offer (3). The fact that this only came out later in the interview does reinforce the notion of the hidden potency of shame. The use of the phrase 'I must admit, right...' (2) suggests Mary feels that this is something to confess. Even when she is acknowledging the fear, she displays very ambivalent feelings, on the one hand agreeing with the phrase I use, that it is 'a big fear' (4) but then saying she does not 'really pay it too much mind' (5):

DJ: Do you think they [professionals] were interested in what you had to say... as someone who knows Rachael?

MG: No they didn't seem to be.... No they didn't seem to be interested.... Do you think that it runs in families? [1] I must admit, right [2], some man, a doctor or other, he was doing a test to see if it ran in families. I've been quite curious about that to be honest, but then again I don't really want to know, I'm curious but I don't want to know – if you know what I mean – because it might play on my mind.

DJ: Someone came to talk to you?

MG: My mum – he wanted to see me and the one after me. Because we've not had any problems.

DJ: Erm... Well, maybe you don't want to know but it's something they're looking into really, that is why that person was interested [3].

MG: Yeah, I was thinking 'oh my god, it may not reach me but if it reaches my child oh my god what am I going to do, you know?' I look at him sometimes and think 'Oh my god I don't want that to happen, I just don't want that to happen'. I don't.

DJ: Is that a big fear?

MG: It is a big fear to be honest, it is a big fear [4], but I don't really pay it too much mind [5]. It is a bit of a fear. Knowing what my mum went through, and what I went through with Rachael and Alison. I wouldn't even want it for Luke [her son], something that I wouldn't wish to happen. Or to me, you know....

There is undoubtedly something *disturbing* about the idea of a genetic link. It will be argued later (in Chapter 6, 'Coping with Stigma: The Significance of Shame and Identity') that this is disturbing for reasons beyond the practical implications. It will be suggested that the idea of genetics makes concrete the psychological identifications people already feel to exist between family members. Talk of, and publicity about, the discoveries of genetic research cause apprehension because they feed into anxieties about selfhood that people already experience. In a significant way, at least unconsciously, it is as though people experience parts of themselves as belonging to or having come from others whom they are close to (notably family members). When those other people become ill, particularly in such a stigmatized way, what impact does that have on their feelings about themselves?

5.4 Madness and a Broken Heart

> Love is merely madness; and, I tell you, deserves as well a dark house and a whip as madness do; and the reason why they are not so punished as cured is, that the lunacy is so ordinary that the whippers are in love too.
>
> Shakespeare, *As You Like It*, Act 3, Sc. 2, ll. 420–6

The hypothesis that was most strikingly different from the biomedical model (Fitzpatrick 1989) was that of a 'broken heart'. This hypothesis supposed that the illness was caused through the person having had relationship difficulties or the trauma of unrequited love. This seemed to be the point at which mainstream psychiatric models departed most from the beliefs of these interviewees. Although stressors are recognized within mainstream psychiatry as being likely triggers of schizophrenic episodes (McKenna 1997, for example), there seems something very specific and poignant about the link that these relatives are making here. The connection between love and madness is hardly new, as the quotation from Shakespeare above suggests. This view of the power and danger of 'carnal love' was also being shared by 'preachers, poets and medical writers' back in the seventeenth century. MacDonald (1981: 88) quotes the medic Burton from this time, who claimed that love turned people 'into very slaves, drudges for the time, madmen, fools, drizzards, abrabilari, besides themselves and blind as beetles'. Interest in links between sexuality and mental health has loomed very large in psychoanalytic theory, of course (Freud 1915; Raynor 1991). Psycho-analysis, however, has become quite marginal to discussions about psychosis within mainstream psychiatry (Clare 1976; McKenna 1997).

The Christodoulou family, for example, thought that George's problems began when he made drastic attempts to lose weight in order to get a girlfriend. Bruce Dear's brother, although not knowing of any specific relationship difficulties that Bruce had experienced, thought that unrequited love offered an explanation:

DJ: What do you think caused it?
MR D: I think he must have been in love with someone, but she left
        him, and he went crazy.... he's never said anything... but
        I think that's what happened. That's what has happened to
        most people who are like that.

There is something that is being considered self-evident here about
a link between love and madness. Perhaps love, or 'being in love' is an
experience that people recognize within themselves as being akin to
madness. Mary Galton also, when asked initially, very firmly saw her
sister's difficulties as being triggered by a split with a boyfriend.

Mike Jenkins is a good example of someone who took quite an open-
minded, eclectic view. Whilst he wondered about ill treatment at the
hands of police (2), he saw the 'trigger factor' for his son's difficulties as
being the traumatic break from a girlfriend (1):

DJ: What do you think caused the illness?
MJ: Well he used to, er... he had a girlfriend. And the girlfriend was
        having an affair with his friend [1], you see. And he tried to
        hurt... you know like lock himself in his room and tried to starve
        himself to death. We had to try and call [the] police to get him out
        the room, he was in there for about three weeks... after that he
        was damaged. One time they arrested him, he told [me] they
        banged his head, they banged his head against the wall [2].

Chris Gyradogc sees his sister's difficulties as being due to a complex
mixture of social and physical reasons. He felt that he and his siblings
were quite socially isolated and stigmatized when young (his parents were
poor Polish immigrants). Chris also remembers that Petra had difficulties with peer relationships at school (1), particularly a close friendship,
which Chris seemed to think perhaps had sexual overtones (2):

... the way that people treated her at that school affected [1] her as
she seemed to be developing quite a good friendship with girls of her
own, I was going to say girls of her own sex but! contradiction in
terms I suppose. But, er, she sort of had a ... it split, you know, she
seemed to be laying a lot on this one relationship, I don't think it was
sexual, I mean maybe it would have developed, but not in that sense –
like a best-friend thing and it just backfired and this friend almost
became her enemy [2]. What she started to do was playing truant from
school, because it's just up the road she used to come home....

Later Chris Gyradogc discusses how he would like to see things develop. He thinks it would be better if his sister lived away from home, which would help her to be less confused about sexuality, amongst other things:

> [I would like] to put her in an independent environment. Where she develops herself basically.... I don't think she has been in that situation, in fact she has never been in a situation where she has lived away from home, she's always lived here [parents' home], apart from the times she's been up in hospital, she has not developed – or had that time to develop certain aspects of her personality. Like her social skills, her sexuality, things like this, I think she's quite confused about quite a lot of aspects – quite a lot of things.

Mrs Karajac thought that unrequited love might have triggered her daughter's difficulties. There seem to have been no particular grounds for thinking this, but again there seems to be something self-evident ('I suppose she must have fallen in love...' [1]. Attendance at a single-sex school is mentioned (2), and further episodes of unrequited love with a nurse (3) and a priest (4):

DJ: What do you think might have caused the problems?

MRS K: All the time that was on my mind. When my sister came she came here four times, the third time when she came my daughter who was about 13, and she came with one of my nephews and she didn't have any boyfriend or whatever, I suppose she must have fallen in love with him [1]. They stayed for three weeks and went back, I remember she suddenly changed, I suppose that must have started it, I don't know. I have a feeling that must be that....

DJ: She was rejected?

MRS K: No but naturally she couldn't go out, she was allowed, she had to work, my husband would say 'Never', in fact at that time if he had accepted that I am completely certain she wouldn't be like that now.... She wasn't allowed to go out and about do,... not allowed to do this or that... all the others used to go out and she couldn't. And she went to a girls' school not mixed [2]. I don't know, all the time I think about that I think maybe that must've been the beginning because when she was in [hospital], she was in [hospital] for one year there was a nurse, an Australian, he was very nice chap, very

> understanding and the first time she was there, [hospital] was very good at the beginning, I must say. So she fell in love with that nurse [3] but he was going to get married and that was the mistake: they should have told her, nobody said it. When the time came for him to go, she became very ill, she did something very bad in hospital, that was when the doctors knew about it, but it was too late. Each time – we are Catholics – there was a young priest she's always attracted to [4] but naturally they put her back in her place and that she doesn't like...because she didn't get what she wanted. I have a feeling that must have been the final thing but now it's too late, I'm sorry to say there's nothing to do about it.

The significance being accorded to romantic relationships is interesting for a number of reasons. It emphasizes the point made in Chapter 4, that the relatives' discourses about mental illness are not simply continuous with modern psychiatric discourses. These lay beliefs do have wide cultural and historical resonance, however. As already mentioned, affairs of the heart had an explicit place in the medical world of early modern England (MacDonald 1981). Chapter 7 will argue that ideas about sexuality and family relationships are still strongly bound up with contemporary notions of sanity and insanity.

5.5   Summary: Placing their Experience within Discourse

The picture that has been painted over the last few chapters is of the family members having recourse to forms of medical model to explain their relative's behaviour. The interviewees' relationship to psychiatric knowledge, and with mental health professionals, is not straightforward, however. The relatives often report poor relationships with professionals and an attitude of some scepticism towards psychiatric knowledge and forms of treatment.

This exploration of relatives' ideas about what caused the 'mental illness' reveals a highly eclectic approach, quite consistent with Furnham and Bower's (1992) study of lay theories of schizophrenia. Individuals are able to hold several parallel, or even contradictory, beliefs. The net was cast wide in the search for meaningful explanations. Certainly the medical model itself was taken up with enthusiasm. Blame and anger could then be safely directed at the illness itself. In addition, other family members might be blamed, or reference might be made to wider social and political events, such as unemployment and police brutality. This is not just a search for meaning, however, but is better characterized as 'a struggle'. It has been argued in this chapter that people's theories were not only shaped by moral concerns of blame and responsibility, but also by powerful feelings of anger, guilt and shame.

One hypothesis that was strikingly at variance with mainstream psychiatry was that which put particular significance on difficulties in relationships, particularly sexual ones. It may be that this reflects a deeply held belief that such relationships are somehow fundamental to mental health, and the understanding (not necessarily conscious) that the observance of sexual boundaries defines mental health in some way. This is an issue that will be returned to in Chapter 7.

Engagement with theories of genetic inheritance, which are fashionable within contemporary psychiatry (McKenna 1997), did present difficulties. For parents, the potentially shameful and guilty feelings that they may have 'given' mental illness to their child are raised. For siblings, the potentially shameful feeling that they are also tainted is aroused. The emergence of these feelings of guilt and shame, often covertly, perhaps under a shroud of aggression, is a very important observation for those interested in understanding the attitudes and behaviour of families. Shame has begun to emerge as an important factor in shaping people's experiences. The next chapter provides a much more detailed exploration of the impact of feelings of shame as we look at families' experiences of stigma and at some of the strategies families may have for coping with these feelings.

6

Coping with Stigma: the Significance of Shame and Identity

The study of the association of stigma and mental illness has a long and distinguished history. To some, the very existence of the concept of mental illness can be understood in terms of stigmatization. There has been an impressive literature on the impact of the label of mental illness on people's behaviour and on the perceptions of others (Goffman 1961; Scheff 1975). Goffman (1963) has noted that the effects of stigma are not confined to those who are directly marked by difference, but reach those associated with that person, referring to this as 'courtesy stigma'. It is very likely that families involved in mental illness will experience stigma (Wahl and Harman 1989). This is a potentially important issue since stigma may well restrict people's willingness to seek help and support (Wasow 1995; Yarrow et al. 1954). In fact, whilst this concern is undoubtedly highly relevant, further exploration of the experience of stigma offers useful insight into the nature of identity and family relationships.

Some people were very open about their experience of stigma. For example, Mr Ajani is quite candid in saying that he does not tell people about his son's difficulties because he feels they would look down on him:

DJ: Do you find it easy to talk to other people outside of the family about what's going on?

MR A: No, not that sort of thing in a society – in my society you don't talk about that sort of thing.

DJ: Why is that?

MR A: Because people would take the mickey out of you, you see what I mean?

DJ: People would look down on you?

MR A: Yeah.

Most interviewees were not so candid about their experience of stigma. It will be argued that this reluctance is a symptom of the influence of shame. The problem people had with talking about issues that involved shame were noted in Chapter 5. It may be that shame is difficult to talk about simply because, as Merrell Lynd (1958: 64) proposes, to do so involves a reliving of those feelings, or, as MacDonald (1998) suggests, people feel ashamed of their own feelings of shame.

Section 1 of this chapter will explore the families' experiences of stigma, emphasizing that these relatives seem to be experiencing stigma by association with their relative.

Section 2 will examine the experience of stigma in more detail, arguing that it can usefully be understood in terms of the emotion of shame. Clausen (1981) argues that the use of the term 'stigma' in relation to mental illness is a gross simplification and needs serious examination. In line with this view it will be argued that there is much to be gained if the experience and the emotions of the stigmatized individual are considered (Scheff 1998). The literature on stigma has largely been based on sociological, or social psychological, perspectives (Lewis 1998). This has meant that the focus has been upon the social processes involved in the formation of stigma, and the consequences of those processes. The emotion of shame has not been studied very much, other than obliquely through the study of stigma, until recently (Gilbert and Andrews 1998). Shame is the feeling invoked in us by what we feel to be inappropriate public exposure, or personal failing. 'Shame is about being in the world as an undesirable self, a self one does not wish to be' (Gilbert 1998: 30). It will be argued that the fact that such powerful feelings were being experienced suggests something important about the strength and nature of the relationships existing between people.

Section 3 will examine some of the strategies that relatives used to ameliorate the effects of stigma and shame. These varied from quite psychological strategies that can be understood in terms of the Kleinian psychoanalytic mechanisms of splitting and projection (Klein 1946), to the more collective response of becoming involved in support groups.

6.1   Shame and the Experience of Stigma by Association

Goffman (1963) gives three classes of stigma: (1) Those involving physical deformities; (2) those comprising blemishes of character involving personal history such as criminal record, unemployment or mental illness; (3) those which attach to groupings of people such as race, nation,

religion or social class. The stigma experienced by the people interviewed here does not quite fit comfortably into any one category. These
relatives are experiencing a threat to their identity (to use Goffman's
term) by association with someone who is seen as mentally ill. Yet, as
some of the following examples will demonstrate, relatives did seem to
feel a very *direct* threat to their own identity, as though their identity
were continuous with the person classified as mentally ill. This aspect of
identity can be understood as operating at both a psychological and a
social level. On the one hand, it can be seen as part of a psychological
process of identification; on the other, it speaks of the social norms and
beliefs that people hold about what it means to be 'related' to someone.
It will be argued that consideration of these people's experience gives
us some insight into the nature of family ties. Here the very distinction
between the social and the psychological realms seems to dissolve: the
more closely the private and intimate worlds of experience are examined, the clearer it becomes that those experiences and the social meanings and constructions of those experiences are inseparable. The
dilemma that these interviewees face is that the person with whom they
are identified is also seen as someone who, in public eyes, is discredited.
The people interviewed experienced parts of themselves to have come
from others; hence when that other person was discredited, so were
they.

When Mrs Peters and Carol Peters are asked about stigma, Mrs
Peters tells first of all of experiences of stigma within the family (1). Carol
suggests that her own acceptance of the situation has reduced her own
feelings of being stigmatized (2). The significance of what 'acceptance'
means will be returned to in Chapter 8. The strategies that people adopt
to cope with stigma will be discussed in the next section of this chapter.
For now it is worth noting the implication that the experience and effects
of stigma are, at least in part, a matter of 'internal' dynamics. Carol is
able to talk more freely about what has happened since she has accepted
that things have changed. Mother (MP) and daughter (CP) then both
angrily compare the large amount of publicity and funding that Aids
has received with the attention given to mental illness. They feel isolated
and neglected. The reference to Aids (3) with its (perhaps shameful)
associations to sexuality and death is surely notable. In spite of the fact
that Carol can talk about having ameliorated the effects of stigma by
reaching an acceptance within herself, some feeling of stigma still persists.

DJ: Yes, often people have difficulty talking outside of the
       family....

MP: Yes, that is quite true, it is still a terrible stigma, there's no doubt about that. I mean I have aunts and things who never mention his name [1]. They never ask after him, they ask after the girls, but they will never ask after him. It is a stigma, yes it is.

CP: Mmm, I find actually myself, I will talk more freely than I did, I have to say, I suppose because after so many years of going through what we've gone through you accept it [2]. And it's just a fact of life, it's there. And so … yes I do talk abut it freely, but I think with certain people you can see a look cross their face because they're not made aware of it, it's not something that, you know there isn't a hell of a lot of publicity about it.

MP: Well we didn't know anything about it, let's face it.

CP: No we didn't, we didn't know anything about it, but also it's not … it's not the sort of thing that's trendy to be part of. Do you know what I mean? I can't explain it, it's just …

MP: Aids is of course [3].

CP: Everybody is going on about how ghastly Aids is.

MP: It is ghastly.

CP: It is ghastly, people are dying of it, but people are also dying. …

MP: Six hundred million pounds was given to Aids at the last …

CP: The trendy charity, everybody is giving to, doing something for Aids and nobody is doing anything for, let's face it, an illness which has been around for centuries. Aids has only just come into being, I mean you know. …

Jason Manula was able to offer further eloquent insight into the nature of the connection that he feels with his brother. In the following extract, when asked about the communication he has with professionals, he tells about how frustrated he feels with professionals who are not responsive, in spite of the fact that he reveals things about himself in order to get them to listen. The strong language (2) that he used when talking about revealing himself to people suggests, certainly anger, but also something else – again perhaps shame – as he attempts to share his experience, to be understood (1):

DJ: Do doctors and other people talk to you about what they think?

JM: Do the doctors? No, not at all. No they don't … you're the first person who has spoken to me about this, and normally when I have taken him to a hospital I have really tried to explain what

it's like [1]. I've tried to, in some cases, even exaggerate a little
but just to make them take notice but, you know, it's so frust-
rating, you know you walk away thinking 'Why the fuck [2] did I go
in there in the first place? Why did I reveal all those personal
things about myself and my family if they're not going to be
responsive?' OK, they have a lot on their plates, that's how
I justify some of their actions but I just....

As the interview with Jason Manula continues, things become plainer.
Jason is very reluctant to reveal himself to others. He does not trust
others with information about his brother. This distrust is not confined
to professionals but is carried through to relationships with non-profes-
sionals. The meaning of the strong language he used becomes clearer.
In talking about his brother he is revealing 'this crap' (1); something
about himself that others may find unacceptable, perhaps something
shameful. Jason's conversation was by no means peppered with strong
language. He swore only twice during the interview, on both occasions
he was referring to self-revelation. Jason also expresses a dilemma that
even though there is danger in self-disclosure, support from others is
seen as essential. Jason feels that the fact that he has less support at the
moment, due to other events in his life (2), has adversely affected his
ability to cope with his brother as he becomes ill this time:

DJ: Have you had people that you can talk to, turn to for support?
JM: Er,...Friends, immediate friends. But even then after a while
      you don't want to encroach on their privacy, you don't want to
      take them for granted. And furthermore they begin to feel 'I've
      heard this crap before' [1]. And also I don't particularly want to
      go to people to relate this same thing year in year out: 'Oh
      another crisis in the family', this type of thing, I mean people
      get fed up. And this time, as I said, I'm going through my own
      personal sort of problems as well, in terms of marriage and
      divorce etc....And I've cut myself off from lots of people. I've
      less people to relate to this time now, at that level [2]. And
      I think that's probably why this time I'm not even taking this ill-
      ness on board.

Jason Manula feels reluctant to talk to others about his brother. He
feels that he is stigmatized. This is an obstacle to his getting the support
which he recognizes helps him cope. Clearly this experience of stigma is
important. There have been strong feelings expressed here involving

not only anger, but also feelings of shame, as implied by Jason Manula's use of strong language and the Peters's reference to Aids. The next section will present the case that the experience of 'stigma' can usefully be understood further by exploring the emotion of stigma – shame.

6.2   Shame: the Emotion of Stigma

Until the 1980s the human sciences had shown remarkably little interest in shame. Even psychoanalysis, which takes the intimate emotions as its subject matter, had been quite neglectful of shame (Giddens 1991; Thrane 1979). Since then there has been growing interest in the effect of shame within psychoanalysis and psychology, and more recently in sociology (Vogler 2000). The chief point of discrimination between shame and guilt is, crudely put, that guilt is about behaviour, shame is about being. Piers and Singer (1953) produced an early formulation of shame, the main themes of which have been developed in the more recent psychoanalytic literature (such as Broucek 1982; Chasseguet-Smirgel 1985; Kingston 1983; Rizzuto 1991). Piers and Singer (1953: 147) distinguish guilt from shame in technical psychoanalytic terms: 'Shame arises out of a tension between the ego and the ego-ideal, not between Ego and Super-Ego.' In other words, shame is the result of a discrepancy between their perception of their actual selves, and their own vision of their ideal self. Guilt, on the other hand, is a perceived discrepancy between actual behaviour and an individual's idea of how they ought to behave. Paul Gilbert, writing from a cognitive and evolutionary perspective, also sees shame as involving this view of the self as undesirable (Gilbert 1998). This conception of shame and its relation to 'ego-ideal' is one that is useful to this analysis. Whilst the concepts of super-ego and ego-ideal were not distinguished clearly by Freud himself (Freud 1923), the distinction has been developed by theorists since then.

Piers and Singer entirely concur with traditional psychoanalytic doctrine (well described by Chasseguet-Smirgel 1985) in arguing that an individual's ego-ideal is made up of:

> the sum of the positive identifications with the parental images. Both the loving, the reassuring parent who explicitly and implicitly gives permission to become like him, and the narcissistically expecting parent and the parent who imposes his own unobtained ideals on the child.   (Piers and Singer 1953: 26)

They go further, however, in claiming that the ego ideal will also be constituted of:

> layers of later identifications, more superficial, to be sure, and more subject to change than the earlier ones, but of the greatest social importance. The 'social role' that an individual assumes in any given social situation, is largely determined by the structure of these developmentally later parts of his Ego-Ideal. There is a continuous psychological interchange between the individual Ego-Ideal and its projections in the form of collective ideals. It is important to recognize the images that go into the formation of this part of the Ego-Ideal do not have to be parental ones at all. The sibling groups and the peer groups are much more significant.   (27)

Parallels with sociological interest in the notion of identity are very clear in the above passage (see Berger and Luckman 1967; Giddens 1991, for example). It is this emphasis on identification and the social nature of those identifications which makes the notion of ego-ideal an important one. It is why Lasch (in the preface to Chasseguet-Smirgel 1985), for example, can argue that this formulation of the ego-ideal 'illuminates...the connections between psychic life and society', or Lowenfeld (1976) that it 'preserv[es] social cohesion probably more effectively than do genuine moral standards'. Scheff (1998) discusses the importance of shame in regulating and maintaining social bonds. Heller (1985) develops a philosophical case for the cultural significance of shame. The social nature of identification and shame is also important in helping to understand Jason Manula's, and the other interviewees', experiences. They feel that not only are their identities made up of parts of other people, but that this identity is continuously constructed through interaction with others. Their dilemma is that a part of their identity is constructed around someone who has, in their eyes and in the eyes of the world, catastrophically altered.

When Jason Manula is questioned more directly about stigma, it becomes clear that the credibility of his own identity is indeed at stake. The feelings of anger and disgust that he has expressed are serving to protect his identity (1) ('image' is the word he uses) from the threat that he feels he faces. Jason feels that he carries around 'traces' (2) of his brother. It is as though there are parts of himself which are his brother. Jason is concerned that the strong image that he would wish to project (3) is damaged by the traces of his brother which he imagines people perceive (4). He feels that others must conclude that he himself has a problem 'deep down' (5). He therefore finds himself avoiding communication about this (6).

DJ: You mentioned feeling embarrassed before. Is it something you have difficulty talking about to some people, you try and hide it?

JM: Yes I think [in] the majority of cases, people who have a similar problem are embarrassed to talk about it.... Yes, it is embarrassing, I don't like talking about it especially to people I don't know very well. And also we all project a certain image [1] out there and once people will connect that flaw with you, they have a certain perception of you. I think some people for example, because when he gets into a very, very bad condition people begin to think that there are traces of you... of him in you as well [2]. When they open the door they look at you very closely to see how you look: are you looking aggressive today or not?!... I mean it's like little subtleties... [edit]. I'm not saying it happens on a large or overt scale but you can see that they seem to think that there is a weak chain in all the sort of image that you project [3] strong, confident, whatever. Because obviously for your brother to be in that condition means that you can't be as strong as all that [4], in that you do have a problem deep down [5] as well and some people want you to talk about it, but you don't want to [6].

Jason feels that people see that there is something lacking about him. This is not stigma simply by association after all, the threat is more direct; part of him is 'weak' because part of him is his brother. Similarly, Ami Brodoff describes the feelings invoked in her by her brother (Andy) suffering from schizophrenia:

I felt that the part of me that was emotionally fragile, that sensed I didn't quite belong, despite belonging, had burst from its boundaries in my inner life and found expression in Andy's illness: What I harbored secretly he expressed to the world.... In his eyes, I saw the disturbing reflection of what I feared I might become. (1988: 115)

6.2.1 Shame, Anger, Sexuality and Identity

The experiences of another sibling can be used to illuminate further the process of identification and its significance to family relationships.

This interview with Mary Galton is one where the effects of 'tainted' identity became very apparent. Her sister's illness has had a dramatic impact on her sense of herself, affecting every aspect of her life including her working life and relationships. When she is asked how her sister's illness has affected her, she describes herself as being on 'edge'. This was not the only interview where this metaphor of being on edge, or living on the edge, is used. Mrs Christian, in Chapter 3, suggests that what she has experienced, and the difficulty that others have in understanding her experience, leaves her 'on the edge of the world'. In Mary Galton's case the words seem to suggest a feeling of nervousness, of frailty, or impending doom; as though the world itself is unsafe or unstable. This can be understood in the context of her family history. Mary's father died when she was quite young. Her mother had emotional problems, as did her younger sister, so when Mary's elder sister became ill, even though Mary was already 22, the impact was still very great. The identification with the older sister seems likely to have been strong. Rachael was her 'big sister', someone who could be depended on.

Understandably, there are practical burdens involved in taking on the role of elder sister (as Brodoff 1988 movingly describes; see also Moorman 1992). There is more to it than this, however. Mary does not visit her sister when she is in hospital. In part there seems to be something unsettling about the hospital itself; 'it's too old, it's too horrible' (2). Perhaps the stigma attached to the hospital, its appearance and the atmosphere resonates too strongly with her own awareness of her threatened sense of herself. She feels the staff look at her as though she is discredited by her association with her sisters (1). There is also the suggestion of there being 'abuse' within the hospital (3). Later this point, about abuse, is clarified when she talks about her sister having to be on mixed-sex wards. Other relatives, too, mentioned this concern; the significance of anxiety about sexual boundaries is discussed in Chapter 7.

DJ: Have you ever felt that, say people at the hospital, staff, were blaming you, or the rest of the family, for what had happened?

MG: Well they did look on us as if to say, you know, 'Oh so you're her sister, oh and your younger sister was in here' [1]. As I say I cannot stand Friern Barnet [hospital], it's too old, it's too horrible [2], the nurses don't seem to care and everything. Whenever I used to go, I did explain to them that,...well I explained to my sisters once they were able to understand, it's not that I don't want to see them: I cannot stand that place.

You know, so I didn't go as much as I should of, 'cos I'm only down the road, but I couldn't take it. I didn't like it at all.

DJ: It was upsetting to see her there?

MG: Yeah, I think ... going back ... that there is a lot of abuse there, I don't have any firm facts, but it's something that I feel and I know there is a lot of abuse in mental institutions [3] ...

DJ: By staff?

MG: Sometimes.... And by other people in there.

It was not only Mary's relationships with professionals, and the psychiatric institutions, that were marred. Mary talked to no one about her sister's illness, not even close friends (1). Then, as she underscores her feeling that she is isolated with the problem of her sister, Mary spontaneously tells a story about her sister being taken to a party by some friends of hers, where she is taken advantage of sexually. It seems as though her friends and the outside world cannot be trusted to look after her sister. It might be argued that this is Mary expressing her own feelings of powerlessness to protect her sister. The concern with sexual boundaries and vulnerability is notable. These are, of course, quite reasonable anxieties to have about her sister. What is remarkable, however, is that the story is spontaneously associated to in response to a question about stigma. There is a visceral quality to Mary's explanation of why she does not talk to anyone else about her sister's difficulties (1). There is something that is experienced as being a part of her: 'It hurts' (2), 'it just feels like a big pain in my chest' (3), the knowledge of her sister's exploitation has broken her heart (4). This visceral language demonstrates how literally, at a subjective level, the identification (incorporation) of others is experienced.[1]

DJ: Is this something you find it difficult to talk to other people about?

MG: Yeah, I don't tell anybody, even my closest friends [1].

DJ: Why is that?

MG: It hurts to talk about it, it hurts [2], so I don't. I don't really discuss it with them.

DJ: What worries you about talking about it?

MG: Even to bring it out it just feels like a big pain in my chest [3]. And some of them people, I know they know Rachael and they've seen what she's been up to ...

---

[1] Bott (1968: 149) discusses how kinship ties can feel very literal in her study of British family and kinship.

DJ: So they know that there is something wrong but you still don't talk about it...

MG: Mmm, I mean like I nearly...two girls I know were up here, and she was desperate to go out and she rummaged in my wardrobe and found a dress and put it on. And somebody said 'Look out of the window', and I saw the two of them taking her out to a party and I knew.... She was on medication at the time and she was drinking, and I told them earlier on, 'Do not, do not, do not, if she comes round here' because one of the girls she was very close with – that was her friend not really mine (it's just they were living close to here). I said to her 'Don't take her out' and it broke my heart [4] to know that she...that they was actually taking her out 'cos I knew they would not be able to look after her and they didn't.... They didn't. For all she knew, all she wanted was a good time, any man could have said whatever he wanted and got what he wanted.... And that is exactly what happened. I didn't speak to them for over a year. I could have smashed their faces to be honest! But it wasn't their fault, I suppose it wasn't really their fault, what could they do?

Mary was a likeable, friendly woman; her talking about feeling she 'could have smashed their faces' was surprising. The aggression is noteworthy (the next section discusses the relatives' use of anger, as a defence against the threat to identity). By this point in the interview, as the extent of the impact that her sisters' difficulties have had on her became apparent, I actually felt quite worried by her sense of distress and isolation. I wondered whether she talks to anyone at all (1). Mary tells me that she has considered getting help for how burdened she feels (2). She finds that forming romantic relationships has become difficult (3) because she feels that her own identity is so tainted (5). She talks to no one outside of the family, assuming that others just could not understand her experience (4). Unlike other interviewees, Mary could not even discuss her sister with others who had similar experiences (6). She sees no prospect of gaining a feeling of solidarity from sharing difficulties with others, such is the degree of the threat of exposure; in her own words, there is something that is 'locked away, shut away: chucked away the keys' (7).

DJ: Do you talk to anyone about it [1]?

MG: No, no, no I don't.

DJ: That's quite a burden then?

MG: Doesn't feel like it. It's been on my shoulders for a long time. . . . Doesn't feel like it. The next thing you'll be suggesting that I need some psychiatrist's help! [laughing]. . . . Well actually I have thought sometimes, . . . I have thought about going to a psychologist just having a sitting-out session of me telling 'em what the hell I want [2]. But I haven't actually got 'round to that. . . . Maybe one day when I've got some money I might do. So someone can listen to me for a change! . . . It's hard, I've cried a hell of a lot, . . . relationships I've had have broken up because of it [3]. I find it very hard . . . um, in relationships to say that my sister has had a breakdown. I've even had relationships at the time when she's having a breakdown for them to even not know that I've got a sister. . . . Because you just don't know what she's going to do or say. . . . And when they've found out, I've told them, when they've found out, they seem to you not to understand, you know.

DJ: The way she behaves?

MG: They can't understand really, can't understand [4] . . . and then they look at me and think 'Well I wonder if she is going to turn out like that?' [5]. In fact that can be a big issue; really a lot of people think that I might have a breakdown or whatever, you know, 'I wonder if she's going to have a breakdown', I don't know. . . . That's why I think I find it hard to discuss it really with anybody. I don't discuss it with anybody. Even at work, we have a temp and her son is going through . . . has had a nervous breakdown and is in hospital at the moment and I wanted to say to her 'I know what you're going through', but it wouldn't come out, it wouldn't come out! [6] And I was like looking at her when she was talking, knowing exactly what she meant but I find it so hard to say: 'Oh, I know what you're going through'. It's just locked away, shut away: chucked away the keys, that's it [7].

Mary went on to say that she felt that her sister's difficulties had interfered with her career as she felt she had not got a deserved promotion because her firm had become aware of her sister's condition. She left the job and was working as a temporary member of staff in another company – 'starting from zilch'. Even her job prospects, she feels, have been adversely affected.

Mary Galton did seem to be in a considerable amount of turmoil and distress, which came over very strongly during the interview. There are powerful and disturbing feelings of anger and shame. She feels that her identity is damaged by her sister's state: her career has been affected, as have her romantic relationships (Secunda 1997 suggests that fear of intimacy is not uncommon amongst siblings of people with mental illness). The chances of her experience being understood by others seemed so slim that it was not worth the further threat to her identity that would be involved in attempting to communicate with others. As will be discussed later on, there do seem to be benefits in talking to others. In not feeling able to do this Mary is left feeling very isolated, confused and vulnerable.

The next section will consider some of the strategies adopted by relatives to protect themselves from the threat to their identity presented by their association with mental illness.

6.3   Defending against the Threat to Identity

It will be argued in this section that there are identifiable strategies that people adopt to protect themselves from this threat to their identity, to ameliorate the feelings of shame. Firstly, the psychological concepts (borrowed from Klein 1946) of splitting and projection will be discussed as a means whereby aggressive feelings can firstly be safely channelled, and then used as part of a withdrawal from the world around them (Craib 1989 and Vogler 2000 discuss these mechanisms, arguing for their social significance). The support that people can obtain from both informal and formal groups, and indeed from their own families, will then be discussed.

6.3.1   Anger: Splitting and Projection

Melanie Klein described the notions of splitting and projection as key psychological processes. Briefly put, these processes involve the disavowal of unacceptably unpleasant feelings, such as aggression, through a number of mechanisms. Splitting involves dividing aspects of the world (including the self) into good and bad, perhaps serving to deny that unpleasant feelings are part of the self, or are part of a loved one. Projection involves the placing of unpleasant feelings onto someone, or something, else (Hinshelwood 1991; Klein 1946).

One could hypothesize that feelings of shame, perhaps mixed with feelings of anger, inadequacy, or even self-disgust (Nathason 1987; Wurmser 1981), may well be projected outwards. If there are feelings of anger and dissatisfaction around people will want to disown these and place them elsewhere. Indeed, we have seen in the previous section that shame appears to manifest itself in quite indirect ways.

As already outlined, the circumstances of the interviewed relatives were such that they were very likely to experience feelings of aggression towards someone who they also construed as a victim, and deserving of care and pity. Thus, a situation of considerable conflict is set up. The mechanisms of splitting and projection would seem to offer solutions. The way that some interviewees talked about fearing their relatives committing suicide, which was discussed in Chapter 3, could also be viewed as a form of projection. By having a fantasy about their ill relative doing themselves harm, their own aggressive feelings could be disowned and projected onto the identified patient.

When Mrs Peters and her daughter Carol were asked directly about their personal experience of stigma (some of their feelings of stigmatization were discussed in the previous section, pp. 94–5), Carol responds quite aggressively: this is surely very defensive laughter she is talking about here (1). Carol appears to use anger to protect herself. The anger she feels is being directed at others; the same fate is 'wished' upon others (2). Carol also seems to be moved to deny the significance of the judgement of the outside world on her. The outside world is belittled. She seems to just stop herself from saying 'what you think doesn't matter' at the end of this passage (3):

DJ: Have you experienced people looking down on you because there is mental illness in the family?
CP: You see I tend to, er... like I'll laugh about it [1], 'So what? I've got a brother with schizophrenia, there are an awful lot of schizophrenics around and that may happen to you!' That's my attitude – 'It could be one of your children or it could be one of your family, it could happen to your brother yet, or your sister', that's my attitude to it now [2] [said quite aggressively].
MP: It isn't mine [softly].
CP: It is mine. Lucinda's [Carol's sister] the same. We laugh. We will openly say 'So what? He's still a person, he's still our brother, we still love him and that's that and what you think doesn't... [3] really doesn't worry me any more, it did but not any more.'

In the passage below, her feeling that it is her brother that needs protecting from the outside world (2), or at least from the adults in it, becomes clearer. Contrast is made with the innocent, non-judgemental child's perception of her brother (1):

CP: But what also comes into play, when he does get like that he'll phone us out of the blue, and if there are other people around and Donald is having an episode, we'll explain to those people that Donald has a problem and then we'll all try and deal with it there. I have to say, I've got a daughter of six and she . . . Uncle Donald is Uncle Donald, children don't see anything like that, which is marvellous about children [1]. [edit] But if there are other people in the house when he comes, . . . I warn them.

MP: Well he doesn't want to meet people.

CP: I do warn them, because I don't want them to make him feel like he's mentally ill. It's not like I'm protecting them, I'm protecting *him* [2] – because I know what he's like and if he feels sort of like this then he'll start acting funny anyway. But if people are normal with him and treat him as sort of my brother Donald then he'll be alright, but I do warn them.

There seems to be a split of sorts. The outside world is derogated to an extent; it is the adults in it that make poor judgements. Thus, the threat to the integrity of their feelings towards Donald is averted. Extracts from another interview will be presented in order to suggest that that anger can be further used to accomplish a withdrawal from the world. Here, the interview itself became an arena where these strong feelings and the mechanism of splitting seemed to be played out.

6.3.2   Anger and Withdrawal

Mrs Land's experiences feature in more detail in Chapter 8 (pp. 138–42) when the particular difficulties she has in coming to terms with her son's circumstances are discussed. Her anger seems to have greater impact than the Peters's above. She appears to employ the anger to derogate and then to withdraw from the outside world. I spent some time questioning her about her experience of stigma. She reacted quite aggressively to being questioned on this issue. Whilst she denied the experience of stigma, she actually disowns any wish to talk to people outside of her family. The number of very idealizing references to family (underlined in the following extract) are interesting and perhaps indicate a degree of splitting. She has split the world into good and bad. Her family is the good into which she has withdrawn, away from the bad outside world. In fact, elsewhere in the interview Mrs Land reveals that her family are not at all sympathetic to Brian and his problems (pp. 139–40), so the family which she describes withdrawing into is a very idealized one. To say that the family she talks of is a 'fantasy' may not be too strong a word. The idea that the ideal or the myth of the family is an important organizing feature of many of these people's lives will be returned to and developed in Chapter 7. Meanwhile, and correspondingly, the 'outside' world is derogated by Mrs Land, it is seen as useless and worthless: 'I'm not interested in other people. I don't find people interesting ...' (1):

DJ: Do you feel able to talk about Brian, to either friends, colleagues...?
MRS L: Only my sister....
DJ: You don't talk to other people?
MRS L: No....
DJ: Why is that?
MRS L: ...I don't have any friends...I only have my colleagues here at work, because I involve myself in <u>my family</u>. I find contentment with <u>my family</u>. I don't need to go out and find someone to talk to because I involve myself with <u>my family</u>, I'm happy, I'm quite happy to go shopping on my own, I do have women who like me to go and see them, I don't want to go, I'm a <u>home-loving</u> person. The only person I'll go with is <u>my sister</u> because we are very close, or I'll go with <u>my daughters</u>, or I'll go with <u>my son</u>, I'm not interested in other people. I don't find people interesting [1] because whether the people I associate with are only interested in talking about themselves. [edit] I can have conversations with them and we talk about different things...but it's very personal to me.... If I spoke to someone who I felt could help me then I would associate with them, I haven't met anyone yet!

Mrs Land seeks to protect her identity by withdrawing and avoiding discussion about what has happened to her son. A process of splitting is discernible: people outside of the family are seen as not good enough to share information with. Kinsella, Anderson and Anderson (1996) note the strategy of self-isolation used by a number of family members they interviewed. To my quite indirect question, Mrs Land (below) denies that stigma has had any impact on her life (1). She does not think, however, that people will understand mental sickness (2). The only person

with whom it is safe to share information is someone else who has had
a similar experience (3). It might be argued that such a person cannot
be a threat because they are similarly threatened, they are in an equal
position (of course, as discussed in the next section, there may well be
positive benefits of sharing things with others).

DJ: Do you think, maybe, that the difficulties with Brian made
         you more private?

MRS L: No, I was always a quiet person [1], ... although I'm happy-
         go-lucky – I'll walk around the office and I'll sing and I can
         talk to people and I can discuss my family with them ... but
         when it comes to discussing a sickness, a mental sickness [2]
         I feel that people don't understand, because they type
         them. ... Unless that person is actually experienced them-
         selves, there is a girl here – she had a nervous breakdown,
         she knows what it feels like, she has a brother-in-law, he had
         a mental breakdown from drink. Occasionally I talk to her
         about Brian because she understands [3], but I wouldn't
         discuss it with ... I found the person that I am able to talk to,
         so I am able to talk to her.

When I ask more directly about stigma, Mrs Land's reaction becomes
quite hostile. Perhaps the vehemence of her denial betrays some insec-
urity. My questions are perceived as being aggressive. In fact I was
aware of becoming more aggressive and almost confrontational at this
point in a way that I avoided in other interviews: I think I was reacting
to defend myself, and in doing so was becoming quite aggressive, and so
became part of that hostile world which Mrs Land withdraws from.[2]

DJ: Do you think people might look at you differently ...
MRS L: No.
DJ: ... if you told them about Brian?
MRS L: No. It doesn't bother me. To me mental sickness, and any
         illness, is an illness to me.
DJ: But I know other people say, they think other people will
         look at them differently, that others will look down on
         them?
MRS L: No. No. I don't feel that at all, I'm proud of my son.

---

[2] This could be seen as an example of 'projective identification', although I have avoided
the term since it is so open to conflicting interpretation (Hinshelwood 1991).

DJ: I know *you* are, but I'm just saying that I know other people have said to me that they are reluctant to talk to friends and colleagues about their son or daughter because they think that they will be looked down on.

MRS L: No. You see I feel confident enough that if I spoke to anyone about my son I'm able to get across to them. Whereas there wouldn't be any of that, I don't believe that people would think that, because I know my own ability that when I start talking to someone they were able to understand. It's just the same to me as explaining to someone how to mend broken bones if I knew how to do it, and that's how I talk to people... I've never found anyone yet, haven't met anyone yet who's been biased. I mean you hear about it, but I've never met anyone. And I feel that if I did meet somebody that I would talk them around it, so that they would understand, so I don't feel that someone's going to think my son's a loony, in layman's language, so it doesn't bother me.

I would suggest that this last sentence ('my son's a loony') rather brutally exposes some of the anxiety that she really feels and perhaps some of the aggressive thoughts that she harbours towards her son, which have been projected onto others. Even in this interview, for a brief period, I become the aggressor, the purveyor of negative thoughts. Perhaps this helps her in her fight to maintain the integrity of her positive feelings towards her son.

This phenomenon of anger being projected outwards and the subsequent withdrawal from the world is one that is likely to be seen by professionals working with families. Its roots as a defence against the anxiety of a threat to identity are worth noting. Strategies adopted by professionals that exacerbated that anxiety (perhaps by appearing to lay blame at the relatives' door) would be directly counter-productive. They would very likely exacerbate the hostility and the withdrawal (Retzinger 1998).

6.3.3 Group Solidarity

The one person that Mrs Land did talk to outside of her family, about her son, was someone who had had similar experiences. Talking to others with similar experiences seemed to be an identifiable strategy used by some relatives. This can be understood as a defence against a threat to identity by associating with those who do not offer a threat. Mrs Dear finds herself reluctant to talk to strangers about her son but, like Mrs Land, she does talk to someone she works with who also has a son with similar problems (1). A measure of how far this seems to set the two of them apart (which suggests a degree of splitting), is given by the turn of phrase used to describe her other colleagues – 'they don't have anything in common with us' (2):

DJ: What about talking about it to people outside of the family, are you able to do that or is it difficult?

MRS D: Most of my friends and people that know me, know that Bruce is not well, I don't hide it from them from the beginning, but to strangers I never really talk to them about it unless I have to, like now you come here I'll talk about it, but apart from that I don't really talk about it.

DJ: Why is that?

MRS D: Um, well partly because I think it is painful to talk about as well, you know, to strangers. If I talk to anyone about it, there is somebody at work – she has got a son who is sick as well like Bruce, and when she mentioned it to me then we can sit and talk about as well, because I think we have something in common and she understands, you know we understand each other [1]. Apart from that I don't see ... I don't know, I don't think they might be interested to listen to us nattering away about our sick son, they don't have anything in common with us [2]. But talking to Ivy, because she has been through the same thing, she's got a sick son so we talk about it.

In this way the experience of stigma is avoided if exposure is restricted to those who have similarly threatened identities. It may also be that such contact with others will offer opportunities to gather information, ideas and build new meanings. Involvement in mutual support groups was a strategy used by relatives and has been recommended in the professional literature (Mannion et al. 1996).

6.3.4 Group Solidarity in Formal Groups

Several people were involved regularly in formal support groups. As Heller et al. (1997) suggest, families are likely to benefit in terms of information garnered, and through the emotional support gained from the relationships in such groups. Wahl and Harman (1989) found that families cited the availability of factual information, and the opportunity for interaction with other families in similar circumstances as the most useful strategies for combating the impact of stigma and isolation. Support groups can provide both of these. Whilst the potential benefits are clear, the preceding sections and chapters should make the point that there are some powerful and perhaps contradictory feelings involved which could create problems. The danger of splitting, with the group being idealized and the outside world being denigrated, being the obvious danger.

Mrs Christian was featured in Chapter 3 (pp. 50–1) talking about how she found difficulty in talking to family because, although they were sympathetic, they could not understand how impossible it was to get over her grief. She found that understanding amongst fellow members of the NSF. It might be argued, however, that this is an example of splitting, the group being idealized at the expense of the rest of the world:

> ...you never have to explain to them how you feel, they know exactly how it feels. They're maybe quite cheerful, but they know...they know it's there, there doesn't have to be any words spoken. They were tremendous. I don't know what I would have done without them. Perhaps family wouldn't be the same because they're emotionally involved in a way.

Perhaps the risk of splitting helps explain Heller et al.'s (1997) negative finding that 30 per cent of the people they studied taking part in such groups reported feeling more overwhelmed and less able to cope after joining a group. It was also striking that groups also seemed to be a source of horror stories about how bad things could get. Perhaps these provided reassurance that there were other people worse off, or it may be that the telling of these horror stories was allowing people to give expression to their own very strong feelings, from the slightly safer vantage point of third-person narrator. Mrs Peters, for example, told me about a 70-year-old couple who were terrorized by their son; or the psychiatric patient who became a paraplegic after a failed suicide attempt. He was then discharged with no back-up or support: 'He's killed himself now, actually. He made quite sure he did it properly next time.'

Jean Karajac was another person interviewed who was involved with voluntary groups. He got information from SANE, which he had heard about through a friend of the family. It was clear that the knowledge he gained was very important to him. He did not attend a support group, but obtained a lot of support from his network of friends, whom he clearly valued. Some of these had knowledge of mental illness from their own degree studies and he found it helpful being able to talk with them.

Mrs Mason was someone who was not inhibited about talking to others; in fact, she would talk to a lot of people about what had happened to her son, finding it gave her a feeling of 'release'. She still found the relatives' group she attended (run by social services) to be very important: it meant that she heard from others in similar situations, realized that she was not alone in facing these difficulties, and gained knowledge.

6.3.5   Big Families, Sharing and Support

Another feature of Mrs Mason's experience was that she had a large and close-knit family around her. They described sharing roles amongst themselves. At times they could alternate roles, give one another a rest if needed. There is some evidence that the outcomes of serious mental illnesses can be rather better in cultures with more extended kin networks (Finley 1998). Certainly it appeared that for some of the interviewed relatives, being in large families seemed to be of considerable benefit. They were able to share information between themselves (group solidarity); they were also able to share practical tasks and burdens. The Cook family, for example, shared and seemed to gain considerable benefit from sharing tasks between them. The Blacksmith family took different roles within the family, allowing Terry to take up a particular new role (discussed in Chapter 8, pp. 144–5) whilst others fulfilled particular expectations, such as having families of their own, having grandchildren and careers.

6.4   Summary

From the previous chapters we know that relatives are coping with a highly complex loss and that they use what is essentially an illness model to explain what they perceive to be the fundamental alteration in their relatives' being. In this chapter the picture of the emotional consequences of having a close family member suffer in such a way has been further developed.

The consideration of the role of the affect of shame is important in elucidating the nature of stigma. It cannot simply be regarded as a social process that operates exclusively outside of, and upon, the individual. For an individual to experience stigma they would not necessarily have had to experience disapproval from others. The discreditation, the discrepancy between how they are and how they would like to be seen, may well exist within the individual. Penny O'Reilly, in attempting to forcefully deny a feeling of being stigmatized as a result of her two brothers' mental health problems, apprehends this dual aspect of stigma. It is how she feels about herself, but also involves feedback from others (1). Her use of the word shame (2) suggests she is not as self-contained as she hopes, and the comment about denying her brothers' existence (3) perhaps betrays some of the strong anxiety she might feel.

> I think you really only experience that sort of feelings of rejection if you feel it yourself. If you feel stigmatized, if you feel that you could be tainted or you think people might think that you're mad as well – that you experience that sort of feedback from people [1], you expect it. If you just say 'I have two mentally ill brothers', people just think 'Oh that's a shame [2], what a tragedy' and that's all, that's the only, the only feedback I've ever had from people: sympathy, pity, er... interest. People might ask questions but er... apart from that no, I've never felt that I wanted to deny that they existed [3].

The shame that people experience depends upon the identifications that exist between people. Analysis of these relatives' experiences suggest that people who are close to us are significant in our lives because we experience them as being a part of ourselves. Such a formulation of the basis for social action as involving essentially irrational processes (Craib 1989; Vogler 2000) is in contrast to the models that assume relations between social actors to be rooted in the rules of economics, such as the principle of reciprocity. Jason Manula's and Mary Galton's experiences of distress through their association with their sibling who suffers from mental illness have been discussed in some detail. It might be understandable if they had simply sought to distance themselves. They have not done this. They have both been very involved in providing and seeking care for their siblings. The explanations that people had for the commitment they felt will be explored in the next chapter. For now, it is worth noting that their commitment might be better understood in terms of the identifications that they experience with their siblings, rather than through any appeal to rational models of behaviour, such as those based on rules of obligation or reciprocity (Finch and Mason 1993). In trying to make good for their sibling they are making good parts of themselves. Their dilemma is that continuing contact with the real, 'discredited' sibling (if they cannot make them well again) will continue to threaten their sense of identity. Brodoff (1988: 115) describes how she felt about distancing herself from her mentally ill brother: 'abandonment of him was an abandonment of part of myself'.

The experience of stigma and the feeling of shame seemed to be important parts of these interviewees' experiences. The very nature of shame makes it difficult to discuss (Merrell Lynd 1958). To admit to feelings of shame in this context would have implications. Not only would it involve the exposure of a most intimate affect but it would also mean acknowledging negative feelings towards the ill person. The issue of the difficulty of coming to terms with such negative feelings is one that will be returned to in Chapter 8.

MacGregor (1994) notes that shame seemed to make people less likely to engage in and make progress through a process of bereavement, and implies that this is due to a sense of guilt inhibiting people from getting over their bereavement. The discussion of shame here suggests a different explanation. Perhaps feelings of shame keep people out of dialogue with others where they might be able to develop new meanings. Perhaps, as Gadamer (1975) has argued, it is only through dialogue that new understandings of the world can emerge. Giddens's formulation of shame directs us to the significance of this withdrawal from dialogue: 'Shame bears directly on self-identity because it is essentially anxiety about the adequacy of the narrative by means of which the individual sustains a coherent biography' (Giddens 1991: 65). Processes of dialogue are very likely to be a crucial means through which those narratives might be repaired. Merryll Lynd also suggests there is something about the experience of shame which implies an immanent concern with meaning:

> Paradoxically, shame, an isolating, highly personal experience is also peculiarly related to one's conception of the universe and one's place in it. Apprehension that one's own life may be cut off from others, empty, void of significance is a terrifying thing, but fear that this isolation is true for others, and that the world itself may hold no meaning is infinitely worse. Experience of shame may call into question not only one's own adequacy and the validity of the codes of one's immediate society but the meaning of the universe itself.
>
> (Merryll Lynd 1958: 56)

Hence the experience of shame has implications for the construction of the meaning of events. Previous chapters have shown how meaning is important in helping people find a pathway through grief. We can now see how shame is linked with grief in the struggle for meaning since the movement through loss requires the building of new meaning (Marris 1978). MacGregor (1994: 163) presents a quotation from a father, describing his feelings of grief over his son's schizophrenic illness, that is highly suggestive of this interweaving of grief, shame and meaning: 'I grieved because I realized that many of my most cherished values were flawed, either in my understanding of those values or in the emphasis I had given them ... I grieved because my longing to see all of life fit into a meaningful pattern has been frustrated. I grieved because I felt isolated from people and alienated from God.'

The next chapter will explore one of the strategies that people use to bring order and meaning to this irrational world of grief, anger, shame and commitment. It will explore the way that the language and imagery of 'the family' is used to structure these aspects of emotional life.

7

The Myth of the Family: 'Love and all that business'

This chapter introduces the metaphor of myth, that is, a story whose premises are not questioned (Barthes 1973; Lévi-Strauss 1968), as a way of exploring and explaining the significance of family relationships. Previous chapters have suggested that relatives of people suffering from mental illness are coping with a range of intense feelings that are often difficult to acknowledge and manage. They are frequently experiencing grief, which is complicated by feelings of ambivalence and anger. Feelings of shame, as discussed in the last chapter, may also be present. Shame impacts on people's feelings of identity and taps into highly sensitive aspects of experience. It will be argued that the notion of family can usefully be regarded as a myth, which brings a degree of order to relationships that are often beset with troubling feelings that are sometimes, although by no means solely, connected to 'sexuality'. The association of the constructs of insanity and *deviant* sexuality has been drawn attention to by many, particularly in relation to ideals of femininity (Chesler 1972; Skultans 1979). Whilst there is, no doubt, some truth in these observations, it will be argued here that there is a highly complex relationship between families, sexuality and sanity. It is not just that aberrant sexuality is sometimes seen as a mark of insanity, but that behaving within the ideals of family is seen as a crucial component of sanity. Chapters 1 and 2 drew attention to the way that some social policies, and mental health policies in particular, have accredited families with great power to psychologically harm or to heal individuals through their styles of discipline and communication. In addition to emphasizing the ideological links that have been made between familial ideals and ideas of mental illness, Chapter 1 also drew attention to historical work that suggested that families themselves were actively using the new categories of insanity and were making use of the asylums. Subseqent chapters have emphasized how active contemporary family members can be in appropriating and using ideas about mental illness.

This chapter will explore how the idea of 'family' is itself very powerful to the family members themselves. It is an idea that not only shapes and constrains notions of sanity but also informs people's hopes for their own lives and their relatives' lives. In accommodating to mental illness, these family members are having to come to terms with the damage that has been done to their own ideals of family life.

Section 1 suggests that familial relationships are beset with mythical ideas because they encompass areas of human life, notably surrounding emotion, sexuality and mortality, that are otherwise hard to include in rational discourse (Brubaker 1984). If the family is a useful rationalization of the troublingly irrational phenomena of sexuality and powerful emotions, then the association between family and insanity becomes unsurprising. Relatives seemed to be using the notion of 'family' as an explanatory device. In searching for explanations for their commitment to relationships that were often painful and (on the face of it) unrewarding, recourse was often being made to the common-sense notion that they were bound together by 'family', or 'blood' ties. In this sense the idea of 'family' can be regarded as a myth. It is a story that glosses over troubling uncertainties and contradictions (Lévi-Strauss 1968; Barthes 1973).

Section 2 explores the impact of the association that is made between ideals of family life and sanity a little further. It is certainly true, as observed by Perelberg (1983a) and Jodelet (1991) for example, that the failure to observe sexual boundaries might be taken as a signal of mental illness. It also emerges that positive engagements with the world of sexuality and romantic/familial relationships were taken as crucial markers and reinforcements of sanity. A significant source of sorrow for the people interviewed was that their ill family member could not live up to those ideals.

7.1 Myth as Explanation

During the interviews with relatives I often found that alongside the considerable admiration I felt at the degree of commitment and the deep concern they showed, I sometimes also felt puzzlement. What kept them involved in a relationship which often appeared to be so painful, which they seemed, on the face of it, to get so little out of? I was most aware of carrying an attitude of puzzlement to the interviews with siblings. Perhaps it is easy to take parents' involvement for granted; parents are supposed to be devoted to their children.

Siblings of people with severe mental illness have not been subject to very much research. One study by Horwitz et al. (1992) looked at the strength and utility of sibling ties when someone suffers from severe mental illness. They view sibling relationships as highly rational enterprises. This rationalism stands in contrast to the experiences of siblings that will be reported here. Horwitz et al. start from a position of concern that siblings will not provide a great deal of support for the patient group, as: '[t]he principle of reciprocity, rather than obligation, may underlie much assistance between siblings so that the flows of assistance run equally between both siblings'. It is assumed that the sibling relationship is a voluntary one, and therefore will only be sustained by mutual benefit. From Horwitz et al.'s standpoint: 'little instrumental advantage emerges for the sibling who provides care for another' (1992: 234). Whilst their data are highly equivocal and suggest that siblings do often stay involved with an ill sibling, there appears to be a hierarchy of obligation operating so that siblings will not provide support in the same way as parents, spouses or children. The most significant point about the study, however, is the assumption that kinship networks function on the exchange of goods and services. These terms have become very common currency within studies of contemporary kinship. Finch and Mason (1993), for example, reported an influential study of family support and helping behaviour in Britain. Its frames of reference provide an exemplary account of the highly rationalistic model of human social functioning (Bendelow and Williams 1998) that is being assumed:

> In much of the existing literature on kinship the concept of reciprocity is a key idea which is used in explaining the foundations of mutual aid in families. It refers to the way in which people exchange goods and services as part of an ongoing and two-way process. Receiving a gift creates the expectation that a counter-gift will be given at the appropriate time. Though reciprocity can take different forms, it is widely seen as being central to the dynamics of kin relations.
>
> (Finch and Mason 1993: 34)

Finch and Mason do, however, see a limit to the usefulness of considering only the negotiation of the exchange of goods and services. They introduce a 'moral dimension' by borrowing Goffman's term, 'demeanour', or social reputation (Finch and Mason 1993: 129). They suggest that material sacrifices might be made in order to maintain an image. There is thus a highly rational process seen to be going on. A calculation is being made with material costs and benefits being considered alongside gains in 'reputation' if people are seen to make material sacrifice. To Finch and Mason, family relationships seem to be based on calculations, material losses are balanced against the positive benefits of enhanced public standing. Parents give gifts to their children in order to 'establish their identities as "generous parents"' (1993: 146). It will be argued here that this is not an adequate model to explain the relationship and commitments that people felt for one another. As described in previous chapters, family relationships often involve highly intense feelings which are often not easy to discuss. What emerges when people do discuss their relationships can be regarded as rationalizations of those feelings wrapped in terms that are usefully thought of as 'myths'.

7.1.1 Myths, Madness and the Family

Lévi-Strauss (1968) suggested that family relationships are embedded within myths because they are concerned with aspects of human life that have become troubling to cultures that put so much emphasis on rationality (Bendelow and Williams 1998). In a nutshell, these troubling aspects revolve around sexuality and mortality. Lévi-Strauss points to the family as the space where biology and culture come face to face. As an example, he argues that the Oedipal myth of Sophocles:

> has to do with the inability, for a culture which holds the belief that mankind is autochthonous ... to find a satisfactory transition between this theory and the knowledge that human beings are actually born from the union of man and woman.   (1968: 216)

He points to the way the Oedipal myth was used by Freud to explain the powerful sexual and rivalrous feelings that Freud believed existed between parents and children. According to Freudian doctrine the infant's introduction to the Oedipal conflict is the point where the child's instinctual drives run up against culture, where society 'enters' the individual and controls and shapes their instinctual drives (see Frosch 1987: 49, for example).

Similarly, Schneider (1980, 1984) argues that the metaphor of myth is crucial to understanding Western kinship. To Schneider the belief that family relationships are special, encapsulated in the mythical idea that 'blood is thicker than water', is such a fundamental truth of Western culture that, like a myth, it is unquestioned (see also Strathern 1992 and Wolfram 1987 for compatible, specifically English, perspectives). Schneider argues that the family fulfils a pivotal role in balancing 'the order of nature on the one hand, and the order of law, the rule of reason, the human as distinct from the animal, on the other hand', bringing the 'two together in a workable, livable human arrangement' (Schneider 1980: 36–7).

Lacan built on Freud's work on the nature of the libidinal (sexual, emotional) ties within families and other groups and argued that such a 'bond of love between members of the church or comrades in arms was established by *discourse*' (quoted in Descombes 1980: 106, emphasis added). In other words, it is discourse, the shared understandings and meanings, which provides the structure that holds people together in groups and societies. That structure, although it may be analysable in rational terms, is itself glued together by forces that are essentially primitive and irrational (in Freudian terms, they are libidinal).

'The family' can thus be usefully regarded as a myth. By this, it is not meant that it is a mere invention, but rather a discourse that offers a means of structuring what might otherwise be alarmingly powerful and arbitrary fragments of emotional experience. Some very troubling feelings, such as loss, shame and guilt, have been explored in the previous chapters. The idea of 'the family' provides something of an *explanation* and a safe container for some of these feelings. To make recourse to the fact of relationships – such as 'he's my brother' – is to provide a gloss over what are otherwise complicated, alarming and irrational feelings.

One particular interview will be discussed in some detail. I was particularly struck, puzzled even, by Mike Harris's attachment to his sister. I therefore spent some time pursuing reasons for his continuing involvement, somehow convinced that there was an *explanation*. Mike had a great commitment to the welfare of his sister, yet they lived very different lives. She periodically spent time in psychiatric wards, psychiatric 'hostels', or sleeping rough in parks. Mike lived in nice house in Barnes (a quite wealthy south-west London suburb). Yet the attachment to Marjorie seemed to have a visceral quality about it, and the concern and protectiveness that Mike extended to both her and her partner Ken was touching.

As a child evacuee, Mike was separated from his parents during the Second World War and his return to London was delayed, such that he was 13 years old before he even met his younger sister Marjorie. Any thought about the significance of early attachment and sibling identification (as in Goetting 1986) had to be revised in this case. There does not seem to have been much reciprocity in material or 'service' terms. The lack of reciprocity in what might be called conventional emotional terms was equally clear: Mike gets no obvious support from Marjorie. I was certainly not given the impression that she was someone Mike would turn to in a crisis. Somehow any notion that he was maintaining face, that he needed to be seen as the sort of person who cares for his sister (Finch and Mason 1993), seems woefully inadequate.

Some detailed extracts from the interview will be presented here to illustrate the way that the search for explanation seemed futile. Mike eventually makes recourse to clichés, such as 'she's my sister'. It will be argued that Mike and other family members seemed to state the fact of their family relationships as though there was something self-evident about them such that further analysis is defied. In this way relations seem to function as though they were 'mythical'.

During the interview itself I used the contrast between his own commitment and the non-involvement of his brother to try and explore his motivation (1). Words like 'obligation' (2) and 'duty' (3) do get used, but the situation is complex. He felt obliged to help his parents as they were elderly; they found it hard to cope with a daughter who could be violent. But his helping entailed the distress of forcing Marjorie back into hospital. These are no dry calculations being made: 20 to 30 years after the events Mike's distress is still tangible:

DJ: Have you any idea what is different between you and your brother that's kept you involved? [1]

MH: Jim's involvement... I think secretly Jim was ashamed of Marjorie.... I mean I'm just, I just had a normal education. Jim did very well, he passed the 11-plus and he went to university and he did very well. And he ... I don't know he, almost wanted to brush... he wanted to brush that side away, it seemed. Um ... and of course I did to some extent have an obligation [2] to my parents, they needed help and ... I suppose it was being duty [3] bound to some extent. Because nobody wants to take responsibility for trying to put anyone in hospital or to enforce – to make her go... in the days just after she had become ill ...

DJ: Was that something that you found quite upsetting?

MH: Yes, absolutely. Because a couple of times it literally became necessary to restrain her because if you ... for instance you'd go into the room and say 'Well Marjorie. We've got to go back now', you'd use all sorts of things to say 'Well if you don't go back now you'll have to go there and you'll never come back again', or 'Your opportunity for coming back at weekends will

go, because...', you know, and even then at times she'd resist
that and it became in the end almost a case of getting hold of
her and taking her to the car. And then she would kick and
punch and swear and it was physical. It literally was physical.
The...hmmmmm...[Mike becomes upset]...and my father
was infirm he just couldn't, he couldn't manage her. And there
was no one else really, I mean who?...You see it wasn't
a police matter, it wasn't...who else to call on...in those
circumstances?

At another point Mike mentions a promise made to his mother:

MH: ...And I always promised my mum that I would – my mum
was absolutely fearful about what would happen to her when
she died...er, and I did promise my mum that I would look to
Marjorie and see what was happening to her.

This point about promises being made to people before they die will be
returned to later in this chapter. Later during the interview, I again
push the question of what keeps him involved, using his own observation of the lack of visitors some people had at the hospital as contrast
(1). He states the fact of the relationship (2), but admits he cannot
really find the words to explain (3) his involvement other than clichés
(4) such as 'love...and all that business' (5):

DJ: What do you think kept you involved, kept you visiting, as you
noticed yourself a lot of people do drop [1]...
MH: Drop off...yeah...um, well...I suppose, she's my sister [2].
It's indefinable [3]...It's something that's there that you...
er...um...the visits did tail off, yes...oh yes...'cos my life
took a turn, my wife's death made a difference...I mean
I could reel off a number of clichés, [4], it's difficult to say why
you go...you say you love her and all that business [5] and you
still do to some extent, there's got to be a spark there...I can't
really elaborate on that one.

And a little later I try again:

DJ: Could you ever imagine dropping out, not wanting to see her?
MH: No, I shall go on seeing her....Yes because I want to. There's
no other explanation or reason...

And yet again a little later Mike still eschews any rational explanation for his feelings for her, despite the fact that she is now so different from how she was and that he doubts she will recover:

DJ: You seem very attached to her?

MH: I am, yes…yes, I am…she's got a…you can't help feeling sorry for Marjorie she's, she's a very caring…she'll always give me a kiss and say…um…she'll say 'I love you Mike'… whether it's, I don't think it's born out of a desire to be, I don't think I'm an insurance policy of sorts, no…it's spontaneous… It's a terrible thing to happen to anyone. Because it's…she's gone from being a bright, nice-looking girl, there's a picture [gets up and gets photo from shelf] that's a school picture – she was quite pretty, when she developed into a young girl of 16, 17 she was very pretty… now…yeah she's let herself go.…It's been a total, total waste of a life. She's had to undergo all that deprivation and…in a way it's worse than…in lots of ways it's worse than death…

DJ: For you?

MH: Well it goes on and on…there seems to be no end. I don't know what the recovery rates are, but I don't think there's hope of recovery…

What is apparent is that for all the probing and questioning, the search for a rational explanation of Mike's involvement kept on hitting a wall. Although Mike Harris raised the possibility of his sister staying involved with him for material gain, even that is dismissed. So far as explanations for his own involvement go, we seem to come up against a wall of what he refers to as 'a number of clichés', such as 'she's my sister', 'love and all that business'. From hearing similar comments in other interviews, I was led to think that I was perhaps coming across the edge of rationality, or the limits of discourse. Perhaps what was being expressed in the exasperation at the lack of words was the feeling that there is a world outside the scope of our rationality, that often there are not words to describe our experience. Maybe what has traditionally emerged to describe the links between people are 'rationalizations' that are summed up by terms such as 'obligation' or 'reciprocity'. Without these rationalizations we are left to fall back on what Mike refers to as 'clichés': 'she's my sister. It's indefinable…it's something that's there that you…you say you love her and all that business…'. Words like 'sister' seemed emblematic of something deeper. After a number of interviews where I met the same 'wall', I began to think of the use of words like family, brother and sister as being used as though referring to something 'magical' or 'mythical' that was invoked to 'explain' what was otherwise inexplicable. For example, in this extract, Sam Mason uses the phrase 'he's my brother' (1), very emphatically. It is a justification of his loyalty to his brother in the face of a society which may not comprehend and in the face of his own acknowledgement that his relationship may be handicapping to himself in certain circumstances:

DJ: Other people often say that they feel that outsiders might look down on them because there is mental illness in the family, has that ever occurred to you?

SM: I don't care, to be honest. I mean initially, possibly ... if you was walking down the High Road and if Charlie had an outburst or whatever, he used to think he was a boxer or whatever, he used to sort of box [laughing] ... or if you're sitting somewhere and he'll start pacing up and down, and initially I was concerned. But then after a while I thought 'Sod it' you know what I mean? OK he's er ... he's MY BROTHER! [1]. He's my brother and it doesn't really matter what other people feel, you know if they had someone and they were physically sick, which is more acceptable to society, then they'd attend for them, they'd look after them and I sort of feel the same. If he's ill then I'll look after him. ... I don't shy away from telling people. I don't really care what people think, I really don't, I don't.

Fred Bryant seems to make a similar recourse to simply stating the fact of his relationship as an explanation of his continuing involvement with his son (1). This is the reason for his giving up his life in the North of England at the age of 60, living with his son firstly in a squat and then an unfurnished council flat:

DJ: What's made you to be so involved? You said yourself before that a lot of families drop out, they can't cope any more, but you've kept going.

FB: Well I suppose ... it's really because he's my son [1], and there are certainly times when I just don't ever want to see him again. There's certainly those times, ... it's like ... to really give you the answer to that, it's like I'm the only one there, there's no one else for John, if I disappear that's it ...

Lévi-Strauss's depiction of parallels between the function of the shaman and the psychoanalyst, observing how they both seek to establish people within discourse, was referred to in Chapter 5 (p. 72). The suggestion being made is that it is very uncomfortable for people to live without a coherent framework of meaning. The ministrations of the shaman and the psychoanalyst (and the counsellor, the social worker, the psychiatrist, or the priest) give meaning and structure to people's experience, which would otherwise remain private, inexplicable and therefore without order and ultimately frightening. For someone to feel that their experiences are beyond discourse, that the social myths (of which family myths are particularly potent) that surround them are no longer coherent, can be extremely alarming. As Mrs Christian described to me (p. 51), she feels as though she is 'on the edge of the world' (and thus produced the sub-title for Chapter 3).

The 'myth of the family' gives meaning to troubling and disparate forces. It might be seen as a useful sack into which the uneasy facets of human experience like love and hate can be placed and kept separate within its own discourse, away from the required rationality of the rest of society. As Busfield (1974: 170) writes of family relations: 'They are subject to a set of ideas, values and beliefs that do not readily corres-pond with those that dominate other social relations ... family relations are one of the few bastions of values that are antithetical to capitalism.'

However, as Roland Barthes protests, myth is not simply a passive vessel into which we can pour our experience but it 'has in fact a double function: it points out and it notifies, it makes us understand something and it imposes it on us' (1973: 117). Myths do more than cover up, myths direct and order us. To Barthes this role of myth carries with it a sinister political function:

> myth is depoliticized speech. ... Myth does not deny things, on the contrary, its function is to talk about them; simply, it purifies them, it makes them innocent, it gives them a natural and eternal just-ification, it gives them a clarity which is not that of explanation but that of a statement of fact. If I state the fact of French imperiality without explaining it, I am very near to finding that it is natural and goes without saying: I am reassured. In passing from history to nature, myth acts economically: it abolishes the complexity of human acts, it gives them the simplicity of essences, it does away with all dialectics, with any going back beyond what is immediately visible, it organises a world which is without contradictions because it is without depth, a world wide open and wallowing in the evident,

it establishes a blissful clarity: things appear to mean something by themselves.   (1973: 143)

Such admonition being attached to myth resonates with critiques of the family, particularly feminist critiques which see the family as a construct which serves to 'naturalize' the patriarchal status quo (Barrett and Macintosh 1982).

On the one hand then, the myth, or discourse, of the family is an important structure to which otherwise troubling feelings can be attached and hence given meaning. On the other hand, it is a force which shapes and constrains, playing an important role in ordering intimate relationships, particularly the sexual mores surrounding those relationships. The next section will explore the implications of this latter point. It will be argued that the ideals of family life were apparent in the way people thought about mental illness and the impact they felt it had on them.

7.2   Family Ideals and Mental Illness

The assumed power of familial/romantic relationships to damage mental health has already been observed. It was noted in Chapter 5 that one theory (held by some relatives) that most jarred with mainstream psychiatric explanations, was that the experience of a romantic trauma could lead to mental illness. The connection between mental illness and sexuality has, of course, been made by others. The observation that has quite commonly been made before is that for an individual to behave in a sexually inappropriate way within a family will lead to the accusation of mental illness (Perelberg 1983a, for example). It would be a mistake, however, to focus only on how madness may be a threat to conventional family life. This would be to ignore how notions of insanity and sanity are positively involved in the construction of concepts about family relationships. It is this point that will be explored further in the following section. It will firstly be argued that the concern with sexual boundaries was not just reflecting anxiety about people with mental illness breaking those boundaries but that there was fear about their vulnerability to sexual exploitation by others. This points to the significance of the respect of those limits themselves. Madness is a threat not simply because it threatens to break those boundaries and assault others but because it does not properly recognize and reinforce those ideals of familial relationships.

The importance of familial ideals could then be seen in the way that the family members interviewed often defined their hopes for the future in familial terms. Envisaging their relative being well and sane was often to see them involved in sexual/familial relationships. In acknowledging this as an ideal, the families were often having to admit that their relatives' illness had done damage to their own ideal of family life. Another clue to the way recourse to notions of family was providing a gloss over the more irrational facets of human experience, was the notable suggestion that some people stayed committed to relatives with mental illness because they had promised parents, before they died, that they would look after the sick sibling. Here the idea of family seems to be used to build a bridge over anxiety about mortality. The presence of madness itself, of course, is a great threat to the hope of continuity that the idea of family offers. There was real awareness of the personal losses that families had suffered in terms of their own familial hopes and ideals.

7.2.1 Sexual Boundaries and Vulnerability

Perelberg (1983a), in her study of families and mental illness, observed that the breaking of sexual boundaries was often the trigger to the 'accusation' of mental illness. The significance of the sexual boundaries between Jacob Doors and his daughter have already been noted (pp. 46–7). He also remembers what made him face the fact that she was becoming disturbed. He recalled her coming home at the age of 15 telling him that a bus conductor had broadcast accusations that she was 'a slut' to everyone else on the bus. It was then he thought 'that someone slightly eccentric was actually hearing voices [and I] didn't quite know how to cope with it'.

Mr and Mrs Snellman reported that one of the first things they noticed about their cousin becoming ill was that he began to imagine he had girlfriends: firstly imagining intimacy between himself and their daughter, and later pestering a young woman where he worked until she made a complaint about him. Mr and Mrs Coles found their son's overt sexual behaviour (bringing home sexually explicit magazines and discussing sexual matters with them) very difficult to cope with. George Christodoulou's sister-in-law felt that he made inappropriate sexualized advances to her, which she found very upsetting and difficult to manage.

Denise Jodelet (1991) studied the difficulties encountered in the integration of a group of psychiatric patients in an 'ordinary' rural community in France. She concludes her study by focusing on the fears which the resident population had about transgressions of sexual boundaries that might occur through their taking psychiatric patients into their families. These fears of 'contamination', she argues, were a major obstacle to integration. Whilst the people I was interviewing did not have, or certainly had not chosen, the option of complete exclusion from 'the insane', there was often a concern with sexual boundaries – as witnessed by the significance given to the rupturing of sexual boundaries in the initial recognition of mental illness. Whilst overt sexual behaviour sometimes appeared as a signal that there were difficulties, there was more often a concern with the vulnerability of their relative; a fear that *they* would be sexually taken advantage of. This is important in that it suggests that Jodelet's (1991) interpretations of people's fear of contamination through contact with insanity need to be considered further. On the face of it, my own observations might suggest the opposite; that these relatives were worried about their own ill relative becoming contaminated by the outside community. Perhaps this emphasizes how the central anxiety is with the observance of the boundaries themselves, rather than necessarily with contamination by what lies on one particular side. Conceivably the reactions of the citizens of Ainay-le-Chateau, studied by Jodelet, are not symptomatic of their fear of insanity itself, but of the way insanity, by definition, does not recognize the boundaries and rules which are seen as necessary to live by. Indeed, it was also apparent that ideals of *successful* sexual and romantic relationships were also prominent amongst the aspirations held by these families.

Mike Harris, as discussed at the beginning of this chapter, for example, became emotional early in the interview as he angrily remembered that his sister had been taken advantage of sexually 30 years earlier. Mary Galton in Chapter 6 (pp. 101–2) presented her angry and emotional description of friends taking her sister to a party where she had been similarly vulnerable. She was also very angry and upset that her sister stayed on a mixed gender ward, where she might be 'abused'.

It was notable that anxiety was also expressed about male sexuality and vulnerability. It did seem that, according to these interviewees, it is not exclusively female sexuality which must be protected or controlled (as Chesler 1972 has prominently suggested). Fred Bryant's sacrifice in moving to London to look after his son can be understood as a reaction to the apparent sexual exploitation his son had suffered in becoming involved in male prostitution. Penny O'Reilly was disapproving of her brother being on mixed wards when he stayed in hospital.

7.2.2 Wishes Framed by Family Ideals

Jason Manula was also worried about his brother's vulnerability when he was not well, as he spent time in a 'red light' district of London and mixed with prostitutes. In contrast to this fear about sexual vulnerability, when Jason Manula describes his brother when he is well he focuses particularly on his ability to sustain a relationship with a girlfriend (1) and behave well towards her. This is perhaps the flip side (to use Jason's phrase) of the concern with sexual vulnerability; that to be successfully involved within a long-term relationship is seen as highly desirable:

DJ: You said he has been quite well for the last couple of years. What has he been like, then?

JM: My brother is a very different person when he's well, he's calm, quiet, loving, considerate, helpful – you name it. It's the flip side of the coin...he's very different when he's well, he's a good communicator, he's fun to be with...um...and he's responsible, very responsible...when he's well, for example in the case of relationships he devotes himself to one girlfriend [1] at the time and he'll give her his all, he'll share his last penny with her, he's that sort of person.

In Chapter 5, it was shown that some people thought that their relative had become ill in response to having been rejected in love. That such theories can be held is testament to the assumed power of intimate romantic relationships. It is perhaps also that the achievement of romantic fulfilment is seen as a very significant goal. This is confirmed by the following sections that refer to the loss of the family ideal, or of the familial aspirations that people hold. The most important manifestation of the ideal of the family was the way in which the relatives' hopes for the ill person were often framed in family terms: having a family of their own, or at least a girlfriend/boyfriend. Perhaps the successful involvement in such relationships is to partake in the rules, to be included in what is seen as an essential aspect of social discourse, to be part of the structure.

Mr and Mrs Snellman, for example, do not, apparently, have to worry about their cousin's financial future, as his grandmother is leaving money in trust for him (1). However, their worries are for his 'purpose in life' (2), in particular, he lacks relationships (3):

DJ: Well, how do you see Erik's future?

MR S: We just don't know, the only thing one can say is that when
        his grandmother dies there should be sufficient money from
        this trust for him to be able to live comfortably [1]. ... But
        that isn't the point, he's got no purpose in life [2], no
        motivation. ... He's had no real personal relationships, no
        girlfriends as far as we know [3].

Mrs Rivers thought the fact that her daughter had always been quiet
may have meant that problems stayed wrapped up inside, causing her
difficulties. Growing through adolescence is seen as a vulnerable
period, when children might become bad, be drawn to crime (1), prostitution and pregnancy (2). Again, it is sexual deviancy which is salient.
She also noted the fact that her daughter did not have a boyfriend
(3), which she felt might have provided her with a reason to get better
(4). To have a boyfriend would be normal, it would be protection from
deviancy:

MRS R: If a person coming out from the children stage, some kids
        coming out from teens, reaching teens, and they turn bad,
        they become really violent thief [1], some come like pros-
        titutes, some have children [2]. It's very hard growing
        up ... you know what I mean? It's a hard life and she is not
        like say she have a boyfriend [3] she has something out there
        to fight to get better for, you see, she don't have nothing to
        fight for [4]. So it's harder with her. ...

Jacob Doors explains that in the past he used to hope that his daughter
would meet a nice man who would look after her and get married (1, 2).
He has now come to the conclusion that his daughter's state somehow,
crucially, precludes such a relationship (3). He explicitly associates
insanity with the inability to love, to sustain relationships:

DJ: What do you think will end up happening to her?

JD: Ohhh, this is one of these things I don't like to face actually.
        Realistically ... when I was younger, a few years ago ... of course
        she's very attractive looking, and delicate, nice voice, I thought
        she might attract a man [1], possibly someone older than her,
        someone of a gentle philosophical nature, sort of person who
        smokes a pipe and wears a velvet jacket. I thought it might
        attract her attention, and get married to her and look after her

[2], that's what I thought, like David Copperfield and his child-wife. She is, however, quite a snappy, difficult person and I think she'd reject David Copperfield and er.... So, er... unless she fell in love with someone who fell in love with her... and looking at it logically I don't think April or someone in her state, I'm talking for all patients: none can fall in love, on a long-term basis. I think love and commitment and all the feeling, they need to come from someone who is sane, if they are not sane they can only love themselves [3]. That's my view for what it's worth, I might be wrong, I hope I am wrong. I don't think so. I don't see, in order to love people you have got to understand people and feel for them, do things for them. If you are tormented by your own problems, there's no way you can understand or feel for another person and anybody that would perhaps spend time with you and try to be kind with you – it might by some sort of peculiar perversion might make you turn on them, I don't know why it should be but I just believe it to be the case. I don't know, I think it would make for tormented relationships one way or the other.

Jacob Doors makes a very positive association between sanity, romance and marriageability. He feels that mental illness somehow precludes people from romantic relationships.

7.2.3 The Damage to the Ideal of Family

Acknowledging that their relatives might not live up to the ideal of engagement in romantic/familial relationships could undoubtedly be distressing in itself. There was also sometimes the realization that their own more personal ideal of what family should mean was damaged. Sam Mason was painfully aware of feeling that he could not take Charlie into his own family (1). This left his brother without a family (2), without the motivation to keep himself well (3):

I'm not sure if we can ever find a solution, sometimes I just accept that it's going to be an ongoing thing because ... we can't take Charlie in, you know, we can't fully take him in to our family [1]....He hasn't got a family of his own [2] so to speak. He hasn't got a relationship so the stimulation and motivation that he needs are not going to be provided [3]. So you sense that he's going to come back to a point where he has to be put back into hospital.

When Jean Karajac reflects on his sister's life, he worries that she will not recover the ground that he feels she has lost. His sister's poor handling of relationships has particular significance. To him, normality would be her being able to have relationships, have a job and perhaps be married. His own feeling of commitment to his sister's future is striking. Somehow he feels his future is bound up with his sister's. His choice of words suggest that he (along with his girlfriend) feels responsible for his sister's future (1). He tried to get a job with the mental health charity and campaigning group SANE in order that his sister might be able to work there too (2). He now hopes that he, with his own girlfriend's help, can do something for her (3):

DJ: Is that how you would ... obviously you would like to see her like that, how hopeful are you that in ten years time she will be like that – in a home of her own with good relationships?

JK: Erm ... I suppose the optimistic side of me says yes – we can do this, we can do that [1]. Like I was thinking if I got the job with SANE then I could have got involved, somehow dragged her to the office, sit her down, make [her] fill envelopes, make the tea or something, make her feel useful [2]. I kept thinking yeah that would be great, I progressed down that line of thought, it didn't happen so it's back to square one. What else can I do to get her involved? Hopefully ... my girlfriend gets along with people pretty well, she's worked for charities herself and I know she's taken some mentally handicapped people away for summer-camp for a week, she's good at people, she's like that ... and somehow she's never been able to get friendly with Janice, I hope that will work out so we can take her out and she'll feel confident, use a bus, she'll gradually become used to interacting with people, that's what I'm hoping [3] ... There again, if the opportunities do not arise then I don't think I can see a future ...

7.2.4   Promises to the Dead

In looking for explanations for Jean Karajac's commitment to his sister we might look to the fact that he was told by his father when he was ill, and dying, that it would be up to him to hold the family together. This may be a very concrete manifestation of people's concern with living up to the ideal of family. Several interviewees mentioned having been asked to look after their ill siblings by parents who were dying. Mike Harris, for example, promised his mother he would look after his sister (see p. 122 this chapter). Kate Daley's mother asked that she and her sisters look after the ill ones. Kate was, however, disturbed that she did not feel she was doing that very well.

On one level, this represents just another example of people struggling to live up to their own ideals of familial behaviour and commitment. On another level, perhaps it hints at something deeper. As Lévi-Strauss (1968) and Schneider (1980) suggest, the myth of the family is being asked to reconcile aspects of human existence, such as sexuality, that do not fit comfortably into Western rationality. Mortality is, of course, another good example of such an uncomfortable fact (Bauman 1992; Giddens 1991). By honouring promises and commitments to the dead, people are in a sense defeating death. Perhaps the idea of family offers the hope of continuity, represented by blood lines and family trees (Borneman 1996; Bouquet 1996).

7.2.5   The Loss of Family Possibilities

For some of the people interviewed, the occurrence of mental illness has robbed them of something that can be understood in terms of a diminution of a family network. Penny O'Reilly expresses very directly how she feels her brothers' difficulties (both being diagnosed as suffering from schizophrenia) have left her, in mid-adulthood, with a diminished (extended) family. The question asked is how she felt her brothers' difficulties affected her parents. The answer quickly comes around to herself and her awareness of how things might have been different. The loss is of the idyll of the extended family, of all the possibilities (1):

> PO: It's a fucking tragedy isn't it, let's face it! I mean...I can't
> ...I can't think how different their life would have been if it
> hadn't happened [sigh, shrugs]. It would be totally different,
> wouldn't it? A totally different life. I mean you'd have two elder
> brothers most probably married with wives and children. It
> would be a different thing entirely. I'd have extra nieces and
> nephews, and two sister-in-laws and a much larger...so you
> think of all the possibilities [1] like that.

Another, particularly sad, example is Mrs Teague who was 73 years old when interviewed. Her husband had died ten years earlier. She does not get on with her other son. Her daughter, who is quite supportive, lives some distance away. Her son, Simon, has become ill and this has left her particularly bereft. She lamented how Simon had been such a good boy, nice, helpful and hard-working. Had he not become ill, 'He would have been my hand and my foot.' Obviously the felt 'loss' of Simon is acute. He would be looking after her now. Instead she feels her future to be very insecure.

7.3　Summary

This chapter has emphasized the very deep attachment that interviewees often felt to their ill relative. Siblings' involvement was notable and striking, despite the fact there have been so very few studies of sibling relationships and mental illness (Horwitz et al. 1992; Horwitz 1993). The role of the maintenance of public identity or even of the exchange of goods and services cannot be ignored as factors influencing family relationships (Finch and Mason 1993). However, the material presented in this and previous chapters surely illustrates that there are other important factors. There are strong irrational feelings involved which are held together within myths, which, as well as giving meaning to our experience, serve to guide and constrain our behaviour. The notion of 'the family' can be justly considered to be such a myth – a myth which, in part, serves the function of bringing a degree of order to the affective ties between people; in particular the troubling world of affect we label 'sexuality'. The concern with sexuality came out in a number of ways. Interviewees showed how the rupturing of sexual boundaries could operate as a signal of difficulties; they also had fears about the sexual exploitation of their relative. The importance of the latter point was indicated by the profoundly emotional way that such fears were brought to my attention. It is also important to note that the positive engagement with romantic, familial and sexual relationships was taken as a crucial marker, and reinforcement, of sanity. It is not simply that mental illness represents a threat to family life, but definitions of insanity are strongly linked to ideals of familial and sexual relationships.

One of the most pressing difficulties facing the interviewees was that, in coming to terms with significant change in their relative, they were also having to come to terms with a seeming violation of the ideal of family. Their lives no longer seemed to fit the pattern of assumptions, of the discourses, which they found around them. The process by which people were able to adapt to this situation and negotiate new relationships will be considered in the next chapter.

8

Managing Myths: Reaching New Understandings

Family relationships are in many ways impossible relationships. They are embedded in myths, and the hopes invested in them can be enormous and might be impossible to realize. What is important is the way that the gap between fantasy and reality is negotiated.

The relatives that have been discussed here have particularly poignant gaps to negotiate between their realities and their hopes and expectations. The many and varied aspects of the relatives' experiences have been highlighted through the preceding chapters. There is the struggle to construct coherent meaning amidst the confusing and frightening series of events. There is the complicated mourning process, the tussle with feelings of shame and the experience of stigmatization. All this takes place within the wider web of feelings, beliefs and expectations that are shaped by, and within, the narrative of 'the family' – to which the presence of mental illness presents such a challenge.

From listening to these relatives it became possible to identify three groups who each took a different view of the current situation. These could be characterized as being different levels of progress along a road towards the acceptance of a changed situation. Whilst it would be wrong to suggest that there is any one correct way of progress, it did seem that the closer to the third level here, the more likely the interviewees were to experience a degree of equilibrium and contentment. The three levels that will be discussed are:

1   An acceptance that there has been an illness operating as an agent of change.
2   An acceptance of the long-term nature of the changes that were perceived to have taken place.
3   An acceptance of *the person* who had emerged from that process of change. This involves the renegotiation of the relationship. A certain amount of spatial and emotional distancing is also, perhaps, inevitable.

This chapter will emphasize the fact that the 'emotional' aspects of people's experiences must be available to be taken into the process of negotiation. The powerful, and often distressing, feelings that people have must take their place in the renegotiation. This is not always easy. Previous chapters have discussed the great ambivalence that is often involved in people's experiences. The common problem was often that this renegotiation of the relationship was difficult when part of the experience of that relationship was being denied or when aspects of that experience are not based on rational judgements and choices, but apparently irrational feelings and impulses. The importance of processes of dialogue emerges very strongly here. Being involved in dialogue with others seemed to be a very important part of the process through which new understandings could emerge. This could be dialogue with other relatives in support groups, with professionals or with the person seen as ill themselves. As Gadamer (1975) implies, it is through dialogue with others that we reach a better understanding of ourselves.

Each of the three suggested levels will now be discussed.

8.1 Acceptance of Illness Construction

As should have become clear by now, nearly all interviewees had come to an understanding of their relatives' behaviour as being due to illness. Mrs Teague and Mrs Lord were the only partial exceptions. Mrs Teague was ambivalent about how she saw things. She told me that she did not see her son's problems as being due to illness (it was the bad company, and smoking), but that she had involved her doctor when Simon started behaving differently. She had not seen her son now for six months. Initially during the interview she was worried that I was there to persuade her to have him live with her. I wonder if, without the firm belief that her son is 'ill', it is difficult for Mrs Teague to cope with some of the very strong feelings she has. The utility of 'illness' as providing a safe target for anger was discussed in Chapter 5. Kinsella, Anderson and Anderson (1996) identified the objectification of illness as being a significant strategy in helping people cope with their feelings of anger. Some support for the importance of the ability to objectify the illness comes from Mallon (2000), who reports interviews with two sisters who had both cut off contact with their mother who had been diagnosed as suffering from schizophrenia. Both of them felt that they could not really separate their mother from the illness, to them she had always been that way. As one sister says: 'Y'see I don't see her as sick, I see her as just my mother. I can't go, "Oh, she had an illness like someone with a broken leg", you know, I just can't do that, it was just...it was all bundled together' (Mallon 2000: 40).

Mrs Lord also did not really see things in terms of illness and blamed the medical system for producing the difficulties her son had. Both of these women had not seen their sons for some time, although neither was really able to discuss the negative feelings that they were perhaps harbouring. It must be said that my understanding of these two people is limited as they did not really engage with the interview. They both felt particularly alienated from the health and social services, which was reflected in their attitude to me. Both were initially very suspicious of my presence, and refused to be tape-recorded. In neither of these people was there a sense of their being engaged in a dialogue, with anyone, through which alternative understandings might develop. My impression was that they were left feeling isolated, upset, angry and possibly ashamed and guilty. The presence of such feelings would be likely to make continuing relationships with their sons extremely difficult. This is perhaps why neither of them had seen their sons for some time.

8.2 The Acceptance of the Long-term Nature of Change, and of the Need for Long-term Support

The next stage of acceptance appeared to be where the long-term nature of the change in their relative is acknowledged, alongside an emerging understanding that they are likely to continue to need long-term support. A form of medical model is implicit to this. Mrs Gazza and her sister-in-law were perhaps typical in being caught in a degree of ambivalence about Mrs Gazza's son. On the one hand, they saw him as someone who needed full-time care for the foreseeable future, but on the other, Mrs Gazza still wondered aloud about brain scans and said wistfully at one point, 'he used to be very kind, a nice boy. I would do anything to make him better. If only it was something like a brain tumour that could be operated on'. The difficulty is here that in *accepting* the long-term nature of the problem, people are also, perhaps painfully, giving up a measure of hope. The dilemma is put well by a parent interviewed by Wasow:

Over a fifteen-year period, we have gone from the totally unrealistic hope for a total cure...to total despair based on our knowldege about the disease and the severe form of it our son has. Now I have no hope left – which enables me to get on with my life, but is the ultimate sadness.   (1995: 161)

Mrs Land is a good example of someone who saw her relative as being changed by illness, but who still clung to the hope that he would be cured. This left her in a painful limbo. She was a woman who seemed to be carrying a great deal of anger around with her. She had a prickly, brittle surface (which emerged during the discussion about stigma – see pp. 106–9). She is angry with professionals, and angry with her family for not doing more. Her son Brian has had very equivocal diagnoses from professionals, although he was certainly very disabled. It was very plain that she carries a dream of curing him. There is painful difficulty in reconciling the way he actually is, and what their relationship amounts to, with what she wishes it to be.

When asked how Brian used to be, her first response is to mention having tape recordings of him as a child (1). Perhaps this, otherwise odd, reference, reflects how solid and fixed is the memory of Brian's old childhood self which Mrs Land carries around. She feels there is no continuity between those memories and the way he is now. His old self is not part of a developing, organic whole, but one that is frozen in time, like a voice trapped on audiotape. Brian is described as a happy, talented child. I am given a quick run-through of his achievements. He learnt to play the guitar, he wrote music (2). He was an electrician, becoming qualified very quickly (3). Then there is his relationship with his mother: the present tense is used, 'he's very close to me' (4), but not to others.

DJ: Did he use to be very different?

MRS L: Oh yes, I've got tape recordings of him as a child [1], he was so happy-go-lucky, joking and he's very, very talented. He taught himself to play the guitar, he's even written his own music [2]. And he went for exams to play guitar, he went for music lessons, he went...he was working, he was working up at [a shopping centre] he was an electrician. He qualified as an electrician within three years rather than five [3]. And yet he was not interested in his school but he qualified as an electrician after 16, and he wrote this music. He even took music lessons with [guitarist], you've heard of him?...So he's not stupid, not a stupid boy, he's very, very sensitive. And he's very close to me [4], but he will react against other people; he says they don't care about him.

Sadly, when asked to expand on their relationship in my next question (1), there seems to be some self-delusion here, an unwillingness to fully face the current situation. These seem to be small scraps of hope and intimacy being gathered up. The description of the shopping expedition is poignant as the significance it is accorded contrasts with the apparent superficiality of the communication between them. The most valuable moment seems to be when he becomes 'his old self' (2), and takes on what sounds to be a child-like role ('What shall we do now, Mum?') (3). Again, it seems to be the past that is being referred to here, a past where he is the child and she is the mother who takes him shopping and buys him clothes. She is also the mother who can look after him and make things better (4).

DJ: So he does talk to you now? [1]

MRS L: Yeh. Uh, I went to see him and all he would say was 'yes, no, I'm alright, don't worry about me', for several weeks and then I arranged to take him out and buy him some clothes and I took him to the shop and all he wanted was a pair of shoes. I took him to the shop and bought him these trainers and when he came out of there for a brief moment he was his old self [2], 'What shall we do now, Mum?' [3], I said, 'Well what would you like to do?' And he said, 'Oh I don't know, anything you'd like to do', so he was back to his old self with me, alone. Then I looked at my watch and I said, 'Oh, it's 5 o'clock, I think you have to get back to the hospital because of your dinner.' He said, 'Yes, I'd think I'd better.' Anyway we walked back, I walked back to the hospital with him...and he said 'Goodbye', and while he was walking through to go into the ward I could see him and several times he turned 'round to see if I was still there or whether he had this feeling he was being watched, I couldn't say... I have a feeling that if I had him home myself, he may begin to improve [4]. ... But living at home with his family, with his sisters and that, I don't think it would work.

A chink in the optimism appears at the end of the passage: she does not really think it would work. When I ask her why not, Mrs Land goes on to give various reasons, why she could not have him home. They were all sensible reasons, no doubt – her daughter and family live with her, and they are not sympathetic to Brian. Her daughter thinks that Mrs Land would not be able to stand the pressure again. These are all factors external to herself – perhaps they protect her from how difficult she finds it to cope with how he really is now. She is able to continue to hope that, in the right circumstances, she will be able to make everything all right: 'when he was on his own with me, he was different'. Mrs Land's own personal myth of her family is protected.

A little later I ask her what effect things have had on her (1). There is more anger expressed at professionals not doing enough. As discussed previously (pp. 106–8), there is a sense that in her anger she is withdrawing into herself, where she can keep control of events (3) (she is referring here to having taken a social worker's advice in asking him to leave her home some years before). At the same time, what is really notable here is that she speaks of guilt (2). Then there is a very sad portrayal of her most recent contact with him, some months ago, when he had visited the family home. It is, however, a sadness which she seemed cut off from. This was presented to me as though it were a pleasant story, a story of hope. Again, it is as though she is trying to get comfort from scraps of intimacy which might reinforce the myth of her family. She again evokes a time when he is the young child and she is the mother (4). Ultimately, however, there is sadness, there is no point in her getting off the bus to talk to him (5).

DJ: What sort of effect has this had on you? [1]
MRS L: Terrible, I worry about my son. I feel guilty about what I've
         done [2] ...
DJ: Guilty?
MRS L: I blame myself for putting my son out on the street. Listen-
         ing to somebody else when I should have followed my own
         instincts [3]. . . . I don't feel that the hospital is doing enough,
         they're doing quite a bit in one sense, they're keeping him
         there . . . Looking after him, he's not on the streets. The last
         time I saw him was a couple, . . . er some months ago. . . .
         Anyway the last time [sigh] he came, he sat down for a while,
         then he went out of the door, five minutes later he came
         back and he started asking me for money. That's what he
         came back for. So I said to him, 'Well, Brian you get an
         allowance'. I said, 'I suggest that you ask the nurse at the
         hospital' (that deals with his money, because he doesn't con-
         trol his own money, she has to give him so much a day, 'cos
         he'll go out and spend it). 'I suggest you go and ask her,
         because you are allowed so much a day.' So he said, 'Oh, all
         right mum', like a child [4], and off he went. And I haven't

seen him since. So whether he's got disillusioned with me again because I didn't give him money, I have the feeling that's it. Occasionally, I see him walking down the street and I'm on the bus. By the time I get off the bus he's way off, gone. So I know there's no point in me getting off the bus [5].

Later Mrs Land talks of the dream she has of making things better. This involves being with him all the time (1), getting the best treatment in a private nursing home (2), treatment that would involve the family and her in particular (3). This dream she has confines her to a relationship with her son in which she assumes full responsibility. Emotionally it is a mothering relationship where he might be a young boy. However, in reality, she is approaching retirement and he is nearly 40:

MRS L: ...if I was rich, if I had lots of money I would do the things for my son that I could do.
DJ: What would you like to do?
MRS L: I would take him out of hospital...I would be with my son all the time [1] and then I would have him taken to a private nursing home, where he would get the best treatment [2], maybe not the best, maybe they are giving him the best now, but...he would get treatment every day, counselling... people that he was able to associate with, people that would be able to bring out his interests through the family so that I could tell them what he likes, what he doesn't like [3]. That way I feel sure that he would be cured, but you've got to have money to do this and I haven't got that sort of money. ...But when I retire, then I'll have the time to be able to try and do something more for him.

Later in the interview Mrs Land reveals a great deal of guilt. She worries that her choice of partner, who was mentally ill himself and violent to her and Brian, had damaged her son. It is in this context that we can see how difficult it would be to accept how different, how 'damaged' Brian now is, because in her own mind she feels responsible for that damage. She feels that the family that Brian was born into was not good enough, that it did him harm. Now she is stuck wanting to fulfil the role of mother, caring and providing for Brian. There is another part of her, however, which seems to realize that she cannot do this. She cannot even have him live with her; she cannot come to terms with the way he is now.

There is no sense of Mrs Land being able to work out a liveable arrangement. She apparently feels great responsibility, guilt and shame (as discussed in Chapter 6). As discussed in the previous chapters, there is likely to be a strong measure of anger being felt towards her son. Those disparate and contradictory feelings remained to be reconciled at the time of interview. It seems as though they cannot be acknowledged; there is no space for dialogue to take place from which a new understanding might emerge. The anger, the shame and the stigma she experiences effectively keep her out of dialogue with professionals, with colleagues and friends, with the rest of her family and even with Brian himself – just as there was no space for dialogue for the two of us to talk about her feelings of stigma (pp. 108–9).

8.2.1 Difficulty in Physically Seeing the Relative

The acceptance of the illness model and of the long-term nature of the change in their relative involves losses. These losses have to be accommodated. Mrs Land is someone who seems unable to face the reality of her son's current situation, so she actually does not go and see him in hospital. Chris Gyradogc seems able to acknowledge that his sister has changed and can talk about it, but has difficulty in accepting her as the person she is now. He lives just a couple of miles from the psychiatric hospital but has not, in over 12 months, visited her there. To see her in hospital would be to face what part of him sees as the 'inevitability' (1) of 'her illness', which is represented all too concretely by the stigmatizing (3) institution. Chris himself suggests that poor communication with the institution and the health authority (2) may be a factor in this situation. Since no communication is taking place, no negotiation of a different understanding of his sister can emerge.

DJ: You mentioned feeling very upset, too upset to visit her [in hospital].

CG: Er...yeah...maybe that's tied in with what I can maybe see as her illness as being an inevitability [1], maybe it's going to go on for the rest of her life. I think I came to the conclusion that it would, you know. Unless something really radical was done, but I don't think, in the foreseeable future, it can be done because of the situation we're in here.... And because we haven't been in communication in an understanding relationship with the institution and the health authority [2]. That's the other thing, the institution is locked up...and the whole idea ... going back to the stigma of the institution [3], it's somewhere where they go and are seen to.

Later, the nature of the difficulty that Chris has in seeing his sister becomes clearer. He has mixed feelings about her returning to live at home, because he would really want the old, 'childhood self' (1, 3) of his sister to come home. However, Chris thinks he is wrong, and that he *should* 'just accept her and her illness' (2).

DJ: How do you feel about Petra coming back here to live?

CG: ...Er...I'd accept it, you know as much as...because I'd have to and that's the way things are, you know. It's just readily accepted...I mean hopefully when she comes back she'll be better, she'll be more calm...so she'll be more pleasant to deal with and she will be more pleasant...so... you know I do miss her, like I do miss...well I miss her yeah, the old her [1]. But maybe that's...er, what I shouldn't be doing, you know, I should just accept her and her illness [2], and not expect her to get well – back to her old self, her old childhood self [3] which I don't think is possible anyway.

On one level Chris Gyradogc knows that his sister has changed; however, on another level, one that might be described as an emotional one, he does have difficulty accepting the person that she is now. So he does not visit her in hospital, and does not look forward to her coming home. To see her in the flesh brings home the contrast between his hopes and expectations and her reality. He does not know what kind of relationship he should have with the real Petra.

There appears to be an important distinction between what people *know* at an intellectual level and what people believe, or feel, at an emotional level. One issue that I have been concerned with highlighting in this book is how important it seems to be for people to be able to incorporate the emotions they experience within coherent systems of meaning. The difficulty is that in order for emotions to be put within discourse they must be acknowledged and brought to the surface.

Mrs Dear is acutely aware of how changed her son seems to her. The awareness, however, is nothing but painful:

DJ: In what way has it affected you, Bruce's illness?

MRS D: [Long pause, tears]...It has affect me a lot, because you know to see how Bruce was, the sort of person he was, and to see him now, he doesn't do anything. Sit around sleeping all day...you know that's the most thing he does now. Compared to how he was he used to like going to work and everything, going off with his friends...he doesn't hardly do anything like that now....So it does affect me because I like to see him the way he was....Not only me anyway, I think it affects his brothers and sister the same that it affects me....

8.3   Acceptance of the New Person and their Role

For some there was acceptance not only of the long-term nature of the change, but also of the changed person. Talk of acceptance, however, must be qualified: it is certainly not a happy acceptance, but more often one of painful resignation and accommodation. It is also important to note that this was a process that, it will be argued, involved the renegotiation of relationships (Secunda 1997 also uses this notion in relation to families coming to terms with mental illness). The renegotiation of the relationships was itself dependent on the development, through dialogue, of a narrative that could be shared within the family.

Elly Blacksmith sees her son Terry as permanently ill and in need of support, if not from her then from her family or professionals. What was notable about this situation was that although she sees her son as needing support, she also identifies a role for Terry. He helps her with household tasks, doing cleaning (1), getting bills paid (2). This appeared to be a very reconciled situation. Perhaps part of this was that he had a role that allowed him, in his mother's mind at least, to be valued for what he did now (even so, she was aware of the loss of the person he had been (3)).

DJ: It's an awful lot for you, obviously.

EB: Yes...not much, because him help me too you know. He go to the shop and do cleaning, sweeping, he do everything for me [1]. He help me very well. Yes he's very helpful like that, he helps me a lot, pay the bills, if I don't want to go to the telephone or to the light or the gas he does it [2]. He helps me a lot, you know, sometimes he takes all my clothes all to the laundry, so you see I would miss him too, [he] takes my clothes to the laundry and he wash and he fold them, he's very good. At least he was a blessed son I would say, growing up he was a very good boy, decent nice boy, but it is a pity you know [3]...and he was bright at school, he went to [a] college, he got a lot of certificates, he passed through college with distinction you know, oh he was so bright, very good....

It should be noted that there were other children in this family whom Mrs Blacksmith regarded as successful. It may be that her own needs as a mother – to have produced a son who was successful, had a job, was married, and perhaps had children of his own – had been met by others. It did also appear that Terry himself is part of that understanding in that he accepted the role he had within the family. Of course, although I did briefly meet Terry, I did not spend much time with him so could not be entirely sure he did not feel otherwise.

It seemed, however, that this acceptance of the current situation was not something that had happened immediately, it had taken time to develop. Mrs Blacksmith has got used to things as they are now (1):

DJ: What effect has all this had on you?
EB: Well I get so used to it, it doesn't trouble me any more [1]....The first time it used to, you know...it used to trouble me a lot, I worry, I fret, I cry...but now it don't matter, it don't trouble me, I only feel sorry of him, the only thing I felt now was sorry,...pity for him, but for myself no trouble me no more because you know you get used to it, from 1980 I think it's time I get used to it! [laughing]. It's full time I get used to it.

8.3.1 Process

There was evidence from other interviews about a process whereby relationships have altered, new relationships have been negotiated. This is an important observation. The development of adult family relationships has received relatively little attention (Cook and Cohler 1986; Greene and Boxer 1986).

Molly Quinn used the metaphor of journey to describe the process which she has gone through in order to reach a position of reasonable equilibrium in her relationship with her sister. She has now arrived (1) at a point where visits are limited to Sundays (2). There was a realization by both parties that visits had to be restricted, but it took years to negotiate (3). The significance of this point will be returned to. It was a long journey, which has not arrived at some simple peaceful place – it is still painful, certainly for Molly Quinn. She still has to cope with negative feelings towards her sister. However, this she does because her sister is family and needs her support (4):

DJ: Some families reach the point where they feel that they can't have much to do with the ill person any more, withdraw – have you ever felt like that?

MQ: Oh yes I have, yes, I've gone through phases where I never want to see her again, but now I've arrived at that level [1]...where she comes down, she's invited down once a week for her dinner on Sunday [2]. Now when I say that, that is a decision that was made that she couldn't come and go because we found it too upsetting and she realizes that too. So we've arrived at a situation where she's very welcome to come down on a Sunday which she does most Sundays, not every Sunday. And then we phone, I phone her almost daily or she phones me. But no I wouldn't want full contact, I can quite relate to that, very much so, and we've arrived a situation where we're both happy on that score, but again it's taken years [3]. Oh yes, I've gone through that phase and even now sometimes if I'm fraught when she rings, I feel 'oh god', you know? Yes I still feel that, but I try to master that for her sake because I feel she doesn't have much in this world, you know, sort of...all she's got is the support of her family which if we withdrew that she would have nothing [4].

An important aspect of the acceptance that Molly Quinn had reached was that she was able to accept having these sometimes very negative feelings towards her sister. After the tape recorder had been switched off, Molly told me that the support of understanding friends had been very important to her. She could say things like, 'I wish she was dead' and not feel guilty, her friends understood what she meant. The likelihood of families harbouring 'dark thoughts' like this was discussed in Chapter 3. For her to be able to admit and understand her own strong negative feelings was surely an important factor in her ability to negotiate a workable relationship with her sister now. For others, renegotiation of the relationship is more difficult whilst those negative feelings remain unacknowledged and thus unavailable to the negotiation.

8.3.2 Renegotiation

This idea of there being a renegotiation of the relationship is a key one. A new relationship has to be negotiated on the terms of the present circumstances. For this to occur, the most relevant factors must be available to be included in the renegotiation. In Molly Quinn's case it was important for her to be able to acknowledge that she had, at times, very strong negative feelings towards her sister.

The Peters family seem to offer a particularly strong example of how this process of negotiation proceeds through dialogue. At interview Mrs Peters and her daughter Carol, whilst as upset as anyone about what had happened, showed a conspicuous affection for Donald, as he was *now*. They talked warmly of his ability at art, and his humour. Whilst still seeing him as being different from the person that he had been, it seemed as though their relationship had developed. What appeared to be critical to this development was a process of dialogue that had allowed an understanding of what had happened to develop between them and with Donald and with the professionals they now had contact with.

Mary Peters and her daughter Carol were interviewed together. There was plenty of sadness about what had happened but the current situation, as it emerged during the interview, had none of the torment that others had. When asked what had kept them involved, Mrs Peters answers in terms that might be seen as duty: 'he's my son' (1). She feels herself stuck in the role of a mother caring for a dependent child until the end of her life. This makes her philosophical about the difficulties she faces: him not wanting to see her and the risk of violence. Carol, Donald's sister, responds differently. To her the crucial point is her own acceptance of the fact of his illness (2). There is no doubt that her brother is different from how he was, but what has happened is bracketed with cancer; it is firmly medicalized. It is also noteworthy that Carol is aware of stigmatizing forces in the world around her (3). However, she says very directly that this stigma does not interfere with what she wants to do. This supplies some confirmation of the idea, discussed in Chapter 6, that to be stigmatized is at least in *part* an internal state. Carol has accommodated to change and difference herself and so, whilst still experiencing 'stigma', she can clearly identify the 'disapproval' of her brother as belonging elsewhere:

DJ: This is maybe a difficult question but what do you think has kept you involved?

MRS P: Well I don't think I'm different from others, from many others, but. . . . Because he's my son and I think it's my duty to be as supportive as I possibly can [1]. And I don't see what else I can do, to be honest with you. When he is appallingly abusive, he doesn't want to see me anyway ... but no, I think you have a son and it's your duty to, er ... support him. I mean as one gets old, this is what worries me, when one isn't able, and we all worry in our group – what happens when we are gone? Because this is the thing that does stick in all our minds.

CP: I think there is another thing as well, that we've accepted that he has a mental illness [2], and that it has to be dealt with like any other illness or if anyone else was in hospital you go and visit them whether it's cancer or a mental illness, and I think, from our point of view, yes we accept there is mental illness and we deal with that accordingly. I think we don't really differentiate between that illness or any other. I mean, you know when I'm in hospital, mummy comes to see me if there is something wrong and I think that probably is also there, apart from being her son, it is also something that you naturally do for a friend or for a brother or for anybody who you know well ... you're not going to get put off by the stigma attached because that is other people's failings, I think [3]. Not ours, not as a unit anyway.

This issue is expanded on later in the interview. Whilst Donald's difficulties are medicalized, there is acknowledgement of their impact. To Carol there is loss in terms the idea of family (1) and what Donald's place in the family might have meant if things had been different. Carol and her mother clearly recognize a fundamental discontinuity between their memories of how Donald used to be and how he is now (2, 3). There is acceptance that things are now different, that it 'will never be the family that it was, ever again' (4):

DJ: Another difficult question, can you say what effect this has had on your life?

MRS P: Oh, shattering actually for all of us, as far as I'm concerned absolutely shattering. I mean it's ... oh, I think it's just about the worst thing that could ever happen really. I mean I think for anyone who has a child who is ill in any way of an extreme nature ... which will never end.

CP: It's like a terminal illness of any kind really. .... You know it's like coping with somebody that's in a wheelchair. One of your children lives in a wheelchair.

MRS P: As far as I'm concerned, I think about him all the time.

CP: Well you think, like all of us, when we think about...when you think about your family you think about the four of us, you don't think about Donald being somewhere else, you just think about all of us as a unit. And, er...I mean...you know my sister and I we sort of...we...I suppose at the beginning you think, 'My god I've lost a brother', because that's what it feels like [1].

MRS P: In fact you have lost him when he's ill....

CP: When he's ill, I mean totally, he's just not there.

MRS P: ...he's not the same at all [2].

CP: You know there's the three of you as children and you've all grown up together, you've all gone to school together...all of a sudden he's not there because he's just...it's a completely different person, it's not the Donald that you know [3]. And as I say you have to accept it in some form or another, but yes, I mean for a mother I would have thought it is the worst thing that can happen is a child being as ill as that. I think it's....It's just a life-long thing really. I mean I think we're all resigned to the fact that this is going to go on for all of our lives and [sigh] we will have to cope with things as and when they come up...

MRS P: Yes, which we do.

CP: And it will never be the family that it was, ever again [4].

Willick (1994) noted the importance of his family reaching 'a painful but better feeling of acceptance' of his son. When I suggest to Mrs Peters and her daughter that 'acceptance' seemed to be important, the point is only lukewarmly agreed with (1). What seems to be felt as even more crucial to them is Donald's own acceptance (2) of his illness status.[1] This, in retrospect, is regarded as a crucial moment in the family's finding a more even keel, and finding they could accept Donald again as 'our brother' (3):

DJ: It sounds as though your accepting of him becoming somewhat different has been important in being able to cope?

CP: Um...yeh, I don't know, I suppose so [1]. Because not that it's important, I just think that is something that you have to do, it's not that it's important, I just think...

---

[1] Fox (1997) describes her acceptance of her own illness as being a crucial step on the road to her 'recovery'.

MRS P: It was when he accepted it, that was a great milestone, when he accepted that he was ill [2], he didn't for a long time....

CP: Yes that's right. He didn't...one's been through so much that...there's so much that's gone through and you tend to feel...'well at what stage did you accept it?' and I suppose we accepted it when he accepted it. It was a big thing for all of us.

DJ: What happened then?

CP: Nothing, he just started talking about it openly.

MRS P: Talking about it openly which he never did before, and he wouldn't accept that there was anything wrong with him.... 'It was all rubbish, everyone was',...I can't remember... 'the doctors were making it all up'...

CP: Yes, that 'They were victimizing him and that work were victimizing him, the company were victimizing him, they wanted to put him somewhere where they wouldn't have to look at him', and all this sort of thing...it was all sort of everybody else....And then all of a sudden he just started talking about the hospital and the fact that he couldn't work and he knew he couldn't work and never would work and that really one's got to look at it like he were an invalid. Remember that, when he was going on about 'really I'm an invalid'?

MRS P: Mmmm...well he does get a disability pension.

CP: Yes...but he wasn't going on about the pension but he was going about the fact that he was an invalid.

MRS P: Well he was quite pleased about that!

CP: Yes, you see this is the thing, you know he's still our brother and that's all there is really [3].

It has been clear in other analyses that a medical model of events is commonly accepted by virtually all the people interviewed. However, what needs to be highlighted here is that what seems to lead this to be a less troubled situation is not just acceptance of the medical model of events, nor just the acceptance of the long-term nature of those difficulties – but the acceptance of the long-term nature of the changes at an everyday emotional level and the acceptance of Donald as the person that he is.

Barham and Hayward (1991), in their study of the experiences of people with psychiatric histories, give prominence to the desire of the people that they talked to, to be accepted 'as people' rather than as mental patients. Barham and Hayward (1991: 139–42) draw on Charles

Taylor's ideas on the construction of modern selfhood. Value and meaning are derived from our ability to construct stories about ourselves, in which we can orientate ourselves within the moral narratives that we find around us.

What the Peters family seem to be telling me here is that they feel they have developed a shared narrative. The family's story is apparently matched by Donald's own, and shared by the professionals they (now) have contact with. They share a discourse, which functions to explain what has happened: why Donald lives as he does, behaves as he does, and why he (to an extent) needs looking after. For the family, there is a coherent web of meaning that holds events together. They are therefore able to relate in a real emotional way (with affection, for example) to the person that Donald is. To Carol Peters, Donald's humour, his art, as well as his strange ideas and occasional violent outbursts, are part of a person that is 'still our brother'. It is important that whilst Donald's illness might be objectified, he is not.

8.3.3   Stepping Back

Another important point about the Peters's situation was that they actually lived in a different part of London from Donald. Generally amongst families where a more stable situation had been reached, there was commonly a belief that there was a limit to how much they could do. This was not a situation that they were going to be able to resolve completely. Specifically, it was realized that they could not live together, as Molly Quinn acknowledged above (p. 146).

Mr and Mrs Snellman had previously been very involved in their cousin's welfare and gone to great lengths at different times to trace their cousin when he had gone missing. When interviewed about their relationship to their cousin, they talked about realizing that they could not cope with being involved as intensively as they had done. They admitted that they were now 'stepping back a bit'. They had now reached a point where they realized there was little they could do when he went away, that they had to get on with their own lives anyway.

Another case that suggests a certain amount of withdrawal is essential if a relationship is to continue is that of Mrs Sutherland, with whom I met twice over a two-year period. Over this time there was a discernible change in her attitude towards her husband. When he first became ill, she had gone to considerable effort to get help for him, trying to get different treatments, visiting specialists and counsellors. She wanted him back to normal. When these strategies failed to work, she had then gone through a period when she could not tolerate seeing him. When I first interviewed her, she had not seen him for about a month and was hoping that he was going to be found somewhere to live well out of the area. Two years on, she had become more accepting of him (although in her terms he was certainly not 'better'). He came to the house regularly and she was glad to see him, pleased to see that he was all right. However, this acceptance of him was on different terms. She no longer had the expectations of him as a husband and they had in fact legally separated.

Those relatives who are unable to accept the long-term nature of change are in a position of conflict, from which they may well want to escape. Jacob Doors was someone who struggled with his daughter's condition and status. He still had hopes which he felt on another level were not realizable: hence some of his strongly conflicting feelings about his daughter. Mr Doors talked about how he had tried to cope with April at home for a number of years. He speaks of the moment of realization that he was not going to be able to continue coping, when he became aware that his daughter did not take the medication unless he physically gave it to her. This was a degree of dependency which he could not really tolerate. He had to give up the idea that she suffered from the sort of illness that was going to be simply mended in hospital (1):

JD: So it was then that I realized, it all came to me, that unless I was physically present she would not take the pills. So that was when I said 'I can't cope', it's me who's taking the pill, not April. I mean [it's like] I've got to take them three times a day, in effect. If I don't do it, then she doesn't, she will stop and she will revert to the state she was then. So then I made it plain – 'Well please yourself, don't take them, I'm not doing it any more' – and then as she deteriorated again then she went... I said, 'I can't cope.'

DJ: You realized she needed full-time care....

JD: Yes, yes, it took some time to work that out. Because before when she went to hospital for quite a while it was like going to hospital – as if you've got something physically wrong with you – you get mended and you come back home [1]. I then realized it wasn't on, I certainly couldn't cope unless I made it a full-time job. If I did nothing else but making sure she took those pills. Seems rather pointless as an existence, for her, for anybody....

Mr Doors was also able to talk about the difficulty of knowing what sort of relationship was appropriate between him and a 27-year-old daughter who had not, in conventional terms, become an adult. He was still looking for the ground on which a new relationship could be negotiated.

8.4 Summary

The relatives have a series of adjustments to contend with in order to reach a degree of equilibrium such that the relationship can continue. The felt loss of the former person has to be come to terms with. There is then the acceptance of the new person that has emerged and the accommodation to that new person. A new relationship has to be renegotiated. A couple of key factors have been identified in this chapter:

1 For renegotiation to take place there has to be a reasonable degree of shared understanding of what is going on. Dialogue is crucial to this process. It can be enormously beneficial if some sort of shared understanding of what has happened can be reached between the ill person and the relative. Additionally, some sort of common understanding of what has happened must develop between the relatives and the outside world (most particularly professionals).

2 People must be able to tolerate having strongly ambivalent feelings towards their ill relative. For various reasons people are likely to experience strong negative feelings towards the ill person. If these are denied it is very hard to renegotiate a liveable arrangement – since some of the vital factors are missing from the negotiation. Feelings of shame, as explored in detail in Chapter 6, may well be very effective in keeping people out of dialogue. Another notable ambivalence was that the achievement of a reconciled new relationship would usually involve letting go of the hope that their relative would be 'cured'. Letting go of such hope was also a loss (Wasow 1995). Of course, one of the difficulties of coping with mental illness can be its unpredictability. Conley and Baker (1990) draw attention to the difficulty some families could experience through the sudden apparent return to health of their relatives.

Throughout this chapter, the theme that has run through the book has become clearer: that people need to be involved in dialogue in order to work out liveable and meaningful solutions. Professionals are often in a good position to facilitate that dialogue, but need to be aware of the ambivalent feelings that families often have.

9

Concluding Discussion: Living with Ambivalence

Carol's Questions

This book began by referring, in the Introduction, to Carol Peters' questions, which she raised during an interview about how she feels about her brother's difficulties:

> How can we deal with this? How are we meant to react? What do you want us to do? ... [C]an you explain to us what is going on in his brain that he is suddenly screaming and shouting at us, and abusing us and everything else, do you know why?

Previous chapters have highlighted the importance of the active 'struggle' for meaning that is going on underneath that questioning and the importance of dialogue in reaching resolution. As Chapters 1 and 2 emphasized, professionals have often approached families with their own rather strong, ideologically informed views that have made dialogue unlikely. For example one reading, or one hearing, of Carol's questions could lead someone to provide answers in terms of practical action. The 'expressed emotion' specialist might suggest the families take a non-critical accepting stance. Leaflets and information might be provided by a psychoeducationalist, outlining the status of current knowledge of neurology, biochemistry or twin studies. Others might see Carol's questions in terms of an unfortunate condemnatory process of labelling. All these responses might, no doubt, have their place, they might perhaps be invaluable. But on their own they would be to miss the point somewhat. Such a simple hearing of the questions would be to blot out the deeper meaning of those questions which can only be understood in the context of the pain and confusion that Carol experiences.

What should have become clear is the importance of the meaning that events hold for the participants. Whilst we cannot prescribe for Carol how she should live her life, what we can do is to listen and understand the difficulties that she faces. A theme throughout the book has been that there was benefit for the interviewees in being able to enter dialogue about their experiences, to put their experiences 'within discourse'. The response of wanting to provide information, to suggest coping strategies (whether based on expressed emotion or any other model) is to present the families with a professional discourse which they may feel excludes their experience.

The attachment and commitment to their relatives, existing alongside the grief, anger and disappointment caused by them, seemed often to be something that simply could not be apprehended by the mainstream models of contemporary kinship that emphasize the rational rules of reciprocity, or obligation. Those relationships, and the ideas people have about mental illness, are importantly shaped by powerful emotions such as love, hate, shame and anger. Some of the causes of these feelings, and the difficulty of coping with the more negative ones, have been discussed. It is likely that the difficulty of integrating conflicting feelings is often compounded by the 'professional' discourse that they find around them, which has largely marginalized the feelings and experiences of families.

Hence there really can be considered to be *a struggle* for meaning. On one level, it is an intrapsychic struggle as individual family members labour with their own conflicting feelings. On another level, they feel themselves to be involved in a fight over whose voice is heard, whose language is used, whose interests, and whose understanding informs the narrative we have about mental illness. It is also important to remember that however much professionals might ignore Carol, her (and her family's) view of mental illness has a major impact on brother Donald's life.

The conclusions of this book can be discussed under three headings. Firstly, it can be argued that families ought to be considered more by those who make and implement policies in regard to people with long-term mental health problems. Secondly, it will be argued that the study points up some quite specific issues for mental health practitioners who may have dealings with families. Thirdly, there are some reflections on the meaning and significance of family relationships and how they can be best studied.

9.1   Families and Mental Health Policies

9.1.1   The Meaning of Mental Illness

The historical evidence gathered in Chapter 1 suggests that families, and ideas about families, have had an influence on the shaping of the broad sweep of policies towards serious mental illness. The historical evidence outlined there portrays families as active participants in the asylum-building process. The evidence gathered from interviews with contemporary families, and presented in Chapters 4 and 5, suggests that families are currently making a contribution to how mental illnesses are understood and responded to. It has been very clear that the relatives interviewed had a strong investment in the medical model of events. This might sit uncomfortably with those that have identified the medicalization of mental distress (Boyle 1990; Laing 1967; Scheff 1975; Szasz 1970) as being a major impediment to progress and understanding. Anyone concerned, however, with the shape of post-asylum policies towards serious mental illness needs to take the families' constructions into account. The findings presented in this book suggest that the medicalization of madness is unlikely to disappear even if the asylums and hospital units are entirely swept away. Analysis of the families' views on mental illness has demonstrated that this view of mental distress is a response to much deeper cultural needs than the professional needs of psychiatrists.

9.1.2   Families as a Resource

As discussed in the Introduction, the difficulties of the group who have been called the 'new long-stay' are salient to any rearrangement in the delivery of mental health services. The group are often portrayed as being rootless, particularly those in more urban areas (Thornicroft, Margolius and Jones 1993). This study, taking place in an urban district of London, suggests that families are often very emotionally involved and can provide a useful resource. They need to be considered by professionals even when they are not living under the same roof as the ill person. Even assuming that there has been a measure of self-selectivity in the families talked to (in that they had agreed to be interviewed), they potentially represent a major source of anchorage for a group of people who often live lives of sad neglect. They are very likely to need support, however, since the emotional toll even when not sharing a household is heavy (the toll on relatives who do share households has been well documented – Brown and Birtwhistle 1998; MacCarthy et al. 1989).

The UK government (DoH 1995; HMG 1999) certainly assumes that partnership between family carers (whether co-resident or not) is highly desirable. Judging by references made in the case-notes and from the reports of the families themselves, professionals barely considered such non-resident families at all. The finding that family members often felt angry and alienated from professionals is consistent with other studies (Creer 1975; Shepherd, Murray and Muijen 1994; Strong 1997). Concerted effort to improve relationships between professionals and families is likely to be necessary. Those concerned with the organization of services could find that the encouragement of training initiatives, aimed at enhancing professionals' understanding of the families' perspective, would enable more constructive work with families.

9.1.3   Living with Mental Illness

Given the seeming importance to families of strategies that involve a certain amount of distancing or stepping back, what of the people who do share a household? The first thing to note is how few people there were still sharing a household (see Appendix B). Only four people at the time they were interviewed were sharing a household. Jane Murray was living in an apparently stable way with her mother. It is perhaps not irrelevant that she was the only person who had recently been in full-time employment, and did certainly have spells where she was clearly functioning very well. The Pickles family also seemed to have reached a position of equilibrium. The Rivers family could be characterized by dogged acceptance and fierce pride in being able to look after their own (perhaps shame as well, not wanting to advertise her illness). She went to a day centre every day, which was undoubtedly important in support. George Christodoulou was living at home, but this was felt by his brother to be an unsatisfactory situation. In addition there was Janice Karajac who, although living with her mother, was admitted during the study period.

Three other people had been admitted to hospital from their family home and it was not clear that they would return home. Mr Jenkins had been living with his son, until his recent hospitalization, but this was not likely to continue. Fred Bryant, whose son was in hospital at the time of interview, felt that he would not be able have his son live with him again. Petra Gyradogc had been in hospital for 12 months and it was not clear whether or not she should return home.

9.2   Implications for Practice: Working with Ambivalence

The study has highlighted a number of aspects of the families' experiences
which, if better understood, might help professionals to work constructively with such families. Greenberg, Greenley and Brown (1997) report
that psychological distress was significantly reduced in families who
experienced a collaborative relationship with professionals. There are
two issues here: firstly, what does this book offer in terms of better
understanding of the families' experiences and, secondly, how might
staff work with these issues?

If families are to be more involved, then they need to be better
understood. This book has emphasized the complex and contradictory
emotions that family members experience. They feel they have suffered
a loss, yet the bereavement process is a difficult one to negotiate. This is
compounded by the involvement of emotions such as shame and the
experience of stigma. All these things have to be woven together in a
cultural ideal of family life.

9.2.1   The Complex Loss

The seemingly most central and common experience was the feeling
that the person they had known, who had become ill, had gone away –
they had become like another person. This defies our normal sense of
the consistency of the self, where we see ourselves and others as, if not
unchanging, at least as consisting of a developing whole (Vaillant 1977).
Many of the relatives' experiences and views can be understood as an
attempt to come to terms with this experience of discontinuity and loss
(Davis and Schultz 1997).

As Freud (1917) highlighted in his classic, *On Mourning and Melancholia*, the bereaved person is coping with the loss of the person that
was, and, more perplexingly, there is the experience of the loss of the
previous possibilities (Willick 1994). When we lose someone close to us
we forfeit something of our own future. For families, parents in particular, these feelings connected to the loss of future expectations they
may have for their children can be terribly poignant.

For some time now, grief has been construed as being the process
through which people accommodate to loss and find fresh meaning
(Murray Parkes 1972). The grief of these relatives, as discussed in
Chapter 3, is complicated by certain features: the fact that the lost
person has not really gone away; the presence of strong emotions, such
as anger, that can be difficult to manage; the stigma and shame of mental

illness (discussed in Chapter 6), which means communicating with others about how they feel can be difficult. There were the additional losses of the often strongly held ideals and expectations of family life that had to be accommodated (as discussed in Chapter 7).

9.2.2 Helping Families Live with Ambivalence

Those families that seemed to have reached a degree of equilibrium (discussed in Chapter 8) were those that had obtained a greater level of acceptance of the person and the situation as it now was. In addition to developing a relationship with their relative on new terms, this involved understanding their own ambivalent and sometimes frankly negative feelings. They were able to let go of the memories and hopes they had and were able to integrate the reality of the person as they now were and move on, rather than simply holding on to memories. In doing this they were letting go of a degree of hope. This is a delicate process.

Ideally professionals would support people through this delicate process. Many studies have now noted the poor relationships that families seem to have with professional mental health workers (Creer 1975; Shepherd, Murray and Muijen 1994; Strong 1997). Such relationships are not likely to be supportive in helping people through that process. There may well be various reasons for the poor relationships. Psychiatric and psychological models that have sought to blame families for causing mental illness might well be influential on many professional perspectives. The overview of the research literature presented in Chapter 2 might well imply that professionals do not have a very good understanding of the families' point of view and their experiences.

Professionals themselves, of course, may well feel 'helpless, angry, despairing and anxious' themselves in the face of mental illness as Spaniol, Zipple and Lockwood (1992:341) suggest. Professionals certainly do feel that they are often excluded from decision making processes, and previous work has drawn attention to the difficulties of managing change in organisations (for example Menzies Lyth 1988). Perhaps more needs to be done to understand the experiences of mental health professionals (Segal 1991, Ramon 1992). Without this work a too prescriptive approach that offered instructions for 'working with families' would seem unwarranted. Given the key role that professionals could play (Spaniol et al. 1992) a couple of suggestions will be made, however.

[handwritten note: prof need to help thru grief to acceptance. Not blame]

9.2.3   Allowing Negative Feelings to be Acknowledged

Given that it may be important for families to acknowledge and come to terms with having very negative feelings, it may be that professionals can make a contribution by encouraging families to express those feelings in a non-judgemental atmosphere.

It may, however, be difficult for mental health workers themselves to endure the apparent ambivalence of the fact that for relatives acceptance of a more pessimistic prognosis can ultimately be more comfortable to live with than continuing to be optimistic. It may run against the grain of their training and outlook, where high priority is given to therapeutic optimism, and encouraging people to higher levels of functioning. Whilst such thinking is laudable and probably helpful, it would still be important for professionals to be aware of the psychological use of such apparent pessimism to the families. Without awareness of this psychological utility it might be easy to see families simply as being involved in a condemnatory process of labelling.

It may be worth reflecting on some experiences I had with families that I was interviewing. On a number of occasions I was given a quite hostile response when I turned up on someone's doorstep. In all cases where this happened, it was possible to overcome this hostility. Allowing space for views to be expressed invariably allowed a more constructive atmosphere to develop. What this suggests is that it is important that professionals, who are working with families in similar situations, allow space for dialogue about ambivalent and negative feelings to be expressed and acknowledged.

Whilst this point is about encouraging reflection, dialogue is something that professionals might consider when working with families. It is important to note that it is not always aggressive feelings that are being hidden, however. Sometimes expressions of hostility can be covering more complex feelings of sadness, guilt and affection. An interview with Penny O'Reilly, who had two brothers diagnosed as suffering from schizophrenia, was noticeable in that it began with her being quite dismissive of them and their lives. The interview changed quite dramatically once the less acknowledged side of her ambivalence had been recognized. For example, near the beginning of the interview:

> I don't think Andrew would benefit from group therapy. He'd bloody bore you to tears! [laughing]. They'd all bore you to tears, honestly, unless people have emotional [problems]. Group therapy helps with emotional [problems] or drink problems, not mentally ill people I don't

think. 'Cos they start talking, bore you to tears about voices and that sort of stuff...um, so I can't see how else they can really help him, apart from medication. He takes drugs. I don't know whether he takes them in tablet form, liquid form, injection, I haven't a clue.

Clearly, a professional hearing this may well conclude that Penny O'Reilly would not make a reliable source of support. However, as I picked up that she was actually more involved than she was letting on (and favourably contrasted this with others), the tone of the interview changed. There immediately followed a long monologue about her involvement and her feelings towards her brothers:

DJ: You obviously do feel quite responsible, a couple of times you've used the word 'ought' about visiting....

PO: I do feel very responsible, they are my responsibility, yep absolutely.

DJ: Where do you think that comes from? Not everyone feels that.

PO: Don't they?

DJ: No, plenty of families eventually give up, cut themselves off.

PO: Oh I think that's...mmmm...it must be because I'm a nice person [laughing]...I can't....I just don't understand why.... Well, I can understand why yes, it depends on the sort of things that they've been up to – I mean you can be at the end of your tether and they can be really nasty and...I'm not saying Andrew or Sean in particular, but I would say that, er...you know you could get one that would come in and beat you up and smash up the house and take your money. You'd want to wash your hands of somebody like that, but, er...I do feel it's my responsibility and a duty as well, I mean – they're my flesh and blood – it's as simple as that and I like them. It just seems strange that people wouldn't do that or would cut themselves off, it's a pleasure – you know if I actually catch Andrew and he's quite funny sometimes it's, you know, it's nice....I mean obviously some parts of it...if you go into his flat, and you see his flat... it's dreadful and that's another duty to go in there and clean it up. I don't do...I'm surprised actually because I feel quite guilty sometimes because I know that I should do more than I do and I don't. And that people can actually cut themselves off entirely is...you know, all credit to them. I wouldn't want to, but when I go to see Andrew sometimes, when I've been admitted into his sanctum – absolute shit-hole of the highest order and

I think 'God' [sighing] and I look around and I think to myself 'I must clear it up', and last time I cleared it up and there were about 12 dustbin bags full of tut. Oh, and the sideboard, and the kitchen and the sink – gunked up. And clothes and shoes,... and people are always giving mentally ill people things, you know, people from the church...clothes, I just bagged up 12 lots of dustbin bags full of rubbish and I'd been to Marks and Spencer and my mother had come over on holiday and we'd bought about a hundred and fifty pounds worth of really nice stuff, you know, trousers, jacket, tee shirts and things like that, really nice stuff. And I felt 'What a waste!' You know in a month's time those things were...but you have to do it, because you should do it and you feel compelled and obliged to do it and you want to do it. You want them to look nice but you go in there and you know that in six weeks' or eight weeks' time they'll be worn to death and just dropped on the floor. You buy... I've gone to his flat and spent money on...oh, washing-up liquid, bleach, scourers, polish, brooms, dustbins, toilet cleaners and various things like that, and you know that they're not going to be used but you buy them hoping that he will use them, that he'll snap out of this stupor and some miracle will occur and the next time you go round to the flat it's going to be clean...but, er,...I do feel that I should do more, in fact. What I really feel like I should do, and if I was a very good person I would do, I'd go round and clean his flat every week, and it would never get in that state, it's only a small thing to do. Here I am living in luxury and he's in squalor and if I could get access to his flat, which is difficult anyway, but if I really wanted to I'm sure I could – actually go in there and clean every week it would only take an hour or two. But I don't, so I'm not that good. I'm not that good at all. I just do.... I suppose in a way I go to see him and to speak to him and, you know, whatever...I go to see him, speak to him and to be with him but in a way I'm as selfish as everybody else because I'm almost by not committing myself to doing that weekly I'm saying, 'But I'm not doing too much – I'm not getting too involved.' So I can understand people cutting themselves off, you know, the nature of some people's mental illness makes them really despicable.

What seemed to happen here was that my commenting on her hidden positive feelings of commitment to her brothers enabled her to talk not only about how committed she did feel, but also her feelings of guilt.

I think the quite brusque way in which she initially describes her feelings for her brothers was covering up a good deal of guilt about how little she feels she does, compared to the affection and commitment that she feels towards them.

There have been many other examples of ambivalence throughout the interview material. The relatives interviewed were able to hold several, parallel beliefs about the cause of mental illness, about diagnosis and treatment. It is important that professionals should be aware of this and be able live with such feelings of ambivalence themselves. Of course, professionals themselves would find this easier if they had good support and supervision.

9.2.4 Encouraging Relative Support Groups

Professionals are being increasingly encouraged to ensure that relatives have access to support and educational groups (Heller et al. 1997; Sheridan and Moore 1991). Such groups have a number of potential benefits, including the gain from feelings of group solidarity (as discussed in Chapter 6) and the accumulation of knowledge that can provide the bases for different understandings to develop. These may have particularly beneficial effects in mitigating the effects of shame and stigmatization (Wahl and Harman 1989), as discussed in Chapter 6.

Whilst the potential benefits are undeniable, there may be dangers in groups (indeed Heller et al. 1997 do find some negative effects). There may be the danger of splitting (Klein 1946), with the groups becoming idealized and the outside world denigrated (as discussed in Chapter 6). This would ultimately have the effect of stifling the communication and dialogue which is so important if new, more reconciled understandings are to be reached.

9.2.5 Ethnic Minority Families

Evidence suggests that support groups may have to be aimed at wider social categories than currently make use of them. Mannion et al. (1996: 49), in reviewing their own and others' evidence on attending support groups, conclude that ways need to be found of attracting 'males, people of low and high income, people with less education, and relatives other than parents'. The importance of sensitivity to ethnic differences and cultural differences (Stueve, Vine and Strueng 1997) in forming groups for different ethnic groups (Finley 1998; Wong 2000) has already been emphasized. Whilst sensitivity is important, unwarranted generalization across 'ethnic' groups is clearly to be avoided. It is clear from the interview material presented in this book that the experiences of being black were often a significant factor in shaping people's understandings (see Chapter 5 particularly). There was evidence that feelings of alienation and mistrust of the psychiatric (and other) authorities were strong amongst many of these black Londoners. However, there were differences in how events were interpreted even within the same family (see discussion of the Mason family, pp. 64 and 78), implying that generalization across cultural or ethnic groups should be regarded with caution (Ahmad 1996; Lambert and Sevak 1996).

9.3 Researching the Family

There is currently a great deal of debate about the decline of the family (Anderson 1994; Laslett and Wall 1972; Robertson Elliot 1996). Figures on divorce, cohabitation, single parenthood and births outside wedlock are held up as evidence of this decline (Poponoe 1988, 1993, for example). Yet the evidence presented in this book suggests that 'the family' seems to be a concept that can carry an enormous weight of significance to people. Such apparent discrepancy is explained by understanding what is meant by the family. The family of 'the family in decline' debate seems to be the functionalist nuclear family limited to the household (Bourdieu 1996). Poponoe (1993: 529), for example, defines the family as 'a group in which people typically live together in a household and function as a cooperative unit, particularly through the sharing of economic resources, in the pursuit of domestic activities'. Although he is careful to include non-married couples, gay families and step-families, this is still a very different understanding of the family from the one that has emerged in this book. Here 'the family' has to be understood in a much wider sense than a domestic space in which children are raised. It was a highly meaningful construct for the adult lives considered here. It could be seen as operating as a myth (Barthes 1973) or a narrative (Plummer 1995), which shapes and orders what are otherwise troubling disparate forces and emotions. The family is not an object that can be measured or counted. It is an idea (Bernardes 1985; Bourdieu 1996; Gubrium and Holstein 1987). Chapter 7 introduced the idea that 'the family' could be understood as 'a myth', that it was a concept that brought order to troubling and disparate forces and feelings. It justifies being understood as a myth because it has become such a seemingly natural object within which certain facets of human experience, which are otherwise very troubling (notably connected to sexuality and mortality), are rendered umproblematic and safe.

9.3.1 Neglected Areas of Family Study

There are a number of quite practical areas that have been neglected through the narrow focus on the nuclear family and the household:

(a) *The study of older adulthood, change and development*

In a sense this book is about how adults are able to develop and accommodate to change within the context of family relationships. Several gaps in traditional research endeavours can thus be identified. Firstly, there has been little work generally on development during the second half of life (Erikson 1982; Guttman 1987; Jacques 1965; King 1974; King 1980; Levinson et al. 1978; Vaillant 1977). Secondly, there is little recognition of the notion of the renegotiation of family relationships over time, particularly as 'children' go through processes of adult development themselves (Greene and Boxer 1986). Thirdly, there has been little work on the reciprocal developmental influences between children (particularly as adults) and parents (Cook and Cohler 1986).

There has been quite a lot of research work covering pregnancy and parenthood as development events (Benedek 1973; Raphael-Leff 1991, for example), but much less on the impact, and developmental aspects, of the experience of having growing and adult children. This neglect is quite consistent with the prevalent psychological and psychiatric model that sees human development as peaking in early adulthood, and then declining from late adulthood. These models have survived in spite of contradictory evidence (Bond, Coleman and Peace 1993; Guttman 1987).

The model presented in this book portrays people involved in struggles to accept and accommodate change and to modify their own expectations. This suggests that more work could profitably be done which examines the psychological development of adult family relationships further.

(b) *The study of adult sibling relationships*

There has been very little work on sibling relationships in adulthood (Goetting 1986; Lamb and Sutton-Smith 1982), yet it has been observed here how strong sibling relationships in adulthood can be (see Chapters 6 and 7 particularly). It is certainly striking that, despite the large welfare and social science industry surrounding the family, for several decades social and behaviourial scientists have lamented the lack of research on adult sibling relationships (Colonna and Newman 1985; Dixon 1997; Greenberg, Kim and Greenley 1997 Lee, Mancini and Maxwell 1990). Certainly beyond childhood, the sibling relationship has been quite neglected by workers in psychology, sociology, or general social science. The evidence gathered by Greenberg, Kim and Greenley (1997), and that presented in this book, suggests that sibling relationships can certainly be a valuable source of support. The relationships themselves can be complicated, however, and they would surely warrant further study.

(c) *The nature of family relationships*

This book has highlighted the influence of shame and the importance of the identifications that people have with each other and with the myths and ideals that they live by. These are important constructs that provide explanations for people's behaviour in ways that traditional models, which assume that people internalize rules or obligations (Johnson 1995; Parsons 1955 and reviewed by Finch 1989), or that they act out of instrumental self-interest, cannot (Finch and Mason 1993). It may be that the observations made here are part of a historical shift. Giddens (1991) for example, argues that shame and its connection to identity is emerging as an increasingly important cultural force that can be seen as a symptom of important historical shift in a 'post-traditional order'. According to this story, family relationships are being governed less according to the rules, obligations and prescriptions of kinship and ever more by the personal relationships built up over time (Giddens 1991; Silva and Smart 1999) and are ultimately dependent upon the irrational worlds of human emotion (Beck and Beck-Gernsheim 1995; Bendelow and Williams 1998; Giddens 1992; Wouters 1992). Whether part of a historical shift or not, it is surely important that more work in the social sciences is able to engage with these worlds.

9.4 Summary: Continuing Conversations

The relatives whose experiences form the foundation of this book have been involved in a series of struggles. They have usually been involved in a whole succession of distressing events through the contact they have with the sufferings of someone close to them. They have also been involved in painful struggle with their own – often alarming and contradictory – feelings of love, hate, shame, anger and despair. They have struggled to fit those experiences and feelings into their own ideals and hopes about what 'family' should mean. They have also faced struggle in finding that their feelings, views and experiences are largely marginalized by the social and professional discourses of mental illness they find around them.

This book has been written as an attempt to address this marginalization. What I have tried to do is to present an honest account of the views and experiences of the relatives so that their experiences might be better understood. An important theme of the book is that new understandings and feelings of acceptance could be reached through processes of dialogue. This book is written as a contribution to a more general dialogue about mental illness. It is not attempting to provide a balanced account of the contemporary world of mental illness. Some of the views presented here, such as the usefulness of the medicalization of mental illness, may be uncomfortable or even offensive to those who see the idea of 'mental illness' as obscuring ordinary human suffering. These differences are not easily reconciled. In mitigation, it is important to recognize that the views held by families about the nature of mental illness are, already, very much a part of the reality in which people with mental health difficulties live their lives. So perhaps, whilst absolute answers about the nature of mental illness may not be reached, the best we can hope for is to develop new and more inclusive understandings. We should continue to have, as Richard Rorty (1980) puts it, conversations that help us to live.

Appendix A: The Structure of the Interviews

The Interviews

The core of the empirical material that forms the bases of the preceding chapters consists of the records of 38 in-depth, open-ended interviews (sometimes with more than one person present), concerning 34 'identified patients'. Letters were sent to families in which a family member had had a long history of contact with psychiatric services in a London Health Authority.[1] The definition of family was simple and pragmatic – it was whomever could be contacted. I tried to make contact with anyone for whom some sort of contact address could be found – very often this was from the 'next of kin' section of medical records. I drew no boundaries around who this might include. It could have been friends, lovers or close relatives. When I made contact with someone, I also always enquired if there were other people involved (and sometimes was put in touch with someone else in the family). For all the potential width of this net, it is striking that I only did one interview with cousins – all the others were with close blood relatives: brothers, sisters, fathers and mothers. I suggest this itself says something significant about the cultural significance of 'blood' relations (Bornat et al. 1999); this issue is discussed in Chapter 7. Details of who was interviewed are provided in Appendix B. Eight of these interviews were not recorded, as a result of either a refusal to be recorded or of conditions not being appropriate for recording.

In addition to relatively formal in-depth interviews, a small number of people (one father, one mother and one wife) were seen more often.[2] This simply allowed for a deeper impression of the impact of events to be gained. The majority of the data and ideas for subsequent

---

[1] All identified patients had at one time had a diagnosis of schizophrenia or bipolar psychosis. Two further selection criteria were used: the identified patient had either had an admission to an acute psychiatric ward for at least six months, or had been referred to the Community Psychiatrist.

[2] A father, Mr Sole, was seen on a weekly basis for around six months and then numerous occasions after that. A wife, Mrs Mansell, was seen on six different occasions. Mrs Mason, a mother, was seen on a fortnightly basis for around nine months.

discussions, however, come from the more circumscribed recorded interviews.

Ethnicity

Seventeen families in the sample can broadly be described as Afro-Caribbean. The sample was drawn from an ethnically mixed urban area of London. Given the over-representation of Afro-Caribbeans in the psychiatric system, these figures are not surprising (King et al. 1994). Asian families were not amongst the sample. This might reflect greater stigma being attached to mental illness, and alienation from psychiatric services amongst those communities (Cinnirella and Loewenthal 1999).

Recording the Interviews

Although most of the people interviewed had no objections to being recorded,[3] it must be noted that four out of the five families who refused to be tape-recorded were Afro-Caribbean. Given the likelihood that this reflects something important about feelings of alienation from psychiatric services amongst ethnic minority groups (Littlewood and Lipsedge 1989), and my presence as a white researcher, these refusals deserve some reflection. Mrs Teague had not seen her son for six months, things had become too upsetting and traumatic. As she relaxed and talked to me it became clear that her only contact with professionals had been when they had been trying to persuade her to have her son back to live with her. It seemed that she assumed I was also there to do that. Mrs Lord was hostile to professionals, blaming them in part for her son's difficulties. I was on the receiving end of that hostility. When it was clear that I was simply there to listen, things became easier. The Cook family were initially hostile and suspicious of my presence. The parents were going to refuse to talk to me, but first got their son to hear what I had to say. He decided it would be all right to talk to me. He and his

---

[3] On two occasions I did not seek to use a tape recorder due to very strong accents (and a felt uncertainty or awkwardness about the interview) and on two occasions there was a lot of background noise. I knew from experience that transcribing is far more difficult than understanding someone sufficiently to converse. Transcription depends on the unaided full comprehension of individual words that are picked up by the tape recorder. In conversation we can get by on the 'gist' of what someone is saying, aided by visual cues.

mother were happy to be recorded, but the father was not. They, as a family, had a great deal of anger for the way that their son/brother had been treated, and for the way that they had been regarded and excluded. Again, the refusal to be recorded seemed to reflect hostility towards the health and social services. I actually spent several hours with them and parted on good terms. These three cases of refusal seemed to be specifically about hostility towards the health and social services with whom I was, in the interviewees' minds, associated.

Mrs Murray was reluctant to be interviewed about her daughter, and only agreed to talk if I just took notes. In her case she seemed to feel a quite strong degree of shame, and even guilt, for what had happened (this is discussed in Chapter 5, p. 81). Whilst we parted on good terms, this was the most difficult interview, with her remaining prickly throughout.

These four refusals have all involved Afro-Caribbean families. The fifth refusal was from a Greek Cypriot family (about George Christodoulou). I interviewed the brother, who did not wish to be recorded. He was initially hostile, saying he did not think he had anything to say. I ended up listening to him for about three hours: about his sorrow about the way his brother was now; about his anger on how little help there had been. He told me that he spoke to no one outside the family about his brother's difficulties. This suggests it may have been something about the shame he felt that made him reluctant to be recorded. The impact of shame is explored in detail in Chapter 6.

Clearly ethnicity may well be a factor in these refusals. Perhaps these families were more likely to feel alienated from services and from me as a white researcher. Certainly the Cook family and Mrs Lord felt that they had been treated differently because they were black. It is worth noting that in all cases I parted on good terms. A bit of sensitivity and a willingness to listen seemed to overcome a good deal of hostility.

Appendix B: Details of Identified Patients (IP) and their Families

Family Name	Relation Interviewed	Accommodation Category of IP	Sex	Marital Status	Age
Ajani	F	3	M	Single	19
Blacksmith	M	4.i	M	Single	32
Bryant	F	2.ii	M	Single	23
Christian	M	2.i	M	Single	42
Christodoulou	B / S-L	1	M	Single	27
Cook	(F/M/B)	4.ii	M	Divorced	42
Daley	S	4.i	F	Single	40
Dear	M	3	M	Single	21
Doors	F	3	F	Single	27
Galton	M/S	4.i	F	Single	29
Gazza	(M/A)	3	M	Single	39
Gouella	A		M	Single	22
Gyradogc	B	2.ii	F	Single	33
Harris	B	3	F	Single[1]	45
Jenkins	F	2.ii	M	Single	29
Karajac	M/B	1 / 2.ii	F	Single	26
Land	M	2.iii	M	Single	33
Light	M	3	M	Single	47
Lord	M	3	M	Single	33
Mansell	W	3	M	Divorced	46
Manula	B	4.i	M	Single	31
Mason	M/S/B	4.i	M	Single	36
Murray	M	1	F	Single	27
O'Reilly	A	4.i	M	Single	37
Peters	(M/S)	4.i	M	Single	35
Pickles	D	1	F	Single	38
Quinn	S	4.i	F	Single	38
Reece	F/S	3	M	Single	28

[1] In long-term partnership with an ex-long-stay patient.

Appendix B   (*Continued*)

Family Name	Relation Interviewed	Accommodation Category of IP	Sex	Marital Status	Age
Regan	(S/B-L)	3	F	Single	38
Rivers	(M/F)	1	F	Single	29
Snellman	C	3	M	Single	33
Sole	M/F	3 /2.iv	M	Single	40
Sutherland	W	3	M	Divorced	36
Teague	M	3	M	Single	37

Abbreviations

M – mother   A – aunt
F – father   C – cousin
B – brother   S-L – sister-in-law
S – sister   B-L – brother-in-law
W – wife   ( ) – only interviewed together.
D – daughter

Accommodation Categories

1   At home with family
2   Hospital at time of interview:
    (i)   long-stay ward
    (ii)   usually at home with family
    (iii)   previously homeless
    (iv)   usually in hostel accommodation
3   Hostel/supported accommodation
4   Independent accommodation
    (i)   Council flat/housing association
    (ii)   DSS-funded bed and breakfast accommodation

Summary of Initial (Identified Patient) Group

Average age = 33   11 women
                          23 men

Summary of Interview Group

15 mothers   8 fathers
8 brothers   8 sisters
Total: 17 men   30 women

References

Ackerman, N. (1958) *The Psychodynamics of Family Life: Diagnosis and Treatment of Family Relationships* (New York: Basic Books).

Ahmad, W. I. (1996) 'The Trouble with Culture', *Researching Cultural Differences in Health*, ed. D. Kelleher, and S. Hillier (London: Routledge).

Alcock, P. (1996) *Social Policy in Britain* (Basingstoke: Macmillan – now Palgrave).

Allderidge, P. (1979) 'Hospitals, Madhouses and Asylums: Cycles in the Care of the Insane', *British Journal of Psychiatry*, **134**, 321–34.

Anderson, K. and Jack, D. (1991) 'Learning to Listen: Interview Techniques and Analyses', *Women's Worlds: The Feminist Practice of Oral History*, ed. Sherna Berger Gluck and Daphne Patai (London: Routledge).

Anderson, M. (1994) 'What is New about the Modern Family?', *Time, Family and Community*, ed. M. Drake (Oxford: Blackwell).

Angermeyer, M. C. and Matschinger, H. (1996) 'Relatives' Beliefs about the Causes of Schizophrenia', *Acta Psychiatrica Scandinavica*, **93**(3), 199–204.

Arieno, A. M. (1989) *Victorian Lunatics: A Social Epidemiology of Mental Illness in Mid-Nineteenth-Century England* (London and Toronto: Associated University Press).

Aries, P. (1962) *Centuries of Childhood* (London: Jonathan Cape).

Atkinson, S. D. (1994) 'Grieving and Loss in Parents with a Schizophrenic Child', *American Journal of Psychiatry*, **151**, 1137–9.

Babiker, I. E. (1980) 'Social and Clinical Correlates of the "New Long-stay"', *Acta Psychiatrica Scandinavia*, **61**, 365–75.

Bachrach, L. L. (1982b) 'Young Adult Chronic Patients: an Analytic Review of the Literature', *Hospital and Community Psychiatry*, **33**, 189–97.

Baker, E. (1997) 'The Introduction of Supervision Registers in England and Wales: a Risk Communications Analysis', *The Journal of Forensic Psychiatry*, **8**(1), 15–35.

Barham, P. (1992) *Closing the Asylum: The Mental Patient in Modern Society* (Harmondsworth: Penguin).

Barham, P. and Hayward, R. (1991) *From the Mental Patient to the Person* (London: Tavistock/Routledge).

Barker, P. (1986) *Basic Family Therapy*, 2nd edn (London: Collins).

Barrett, M. and Macintosh, M. (1982) *The Anti-Social Family* (London: Verso).

Barthes, R. (1973) *Mythologies*, trans. Annette Lavers (London: Paladin Books).

Bartlett, P. and Wright, D. (1999) *Outside the Walls of the Asylum: The History of Commuity Care, 1750–2000* (London: The Athlone Press).

Barton, N. (1959) *Institutional Neurosis* (London: Wright).

Bateson, G., Jackson, D., Haley, J. and Weakland, J. (1955) 'Towards a Theory of Schizophrenia', *Behaviourial Science*, **1**.

Baumam, Z. (1992) *Mortality and Immortality and Other Life Strategies* (Cambridge: Polity Press).

Beck, U. and Beck-Gernsheim, E. (1995) *The Normal Chaos of Love*, trans. M. Ritter and J. Wiebel (Cambridge: Polity Press).

Bendelow, G. and Williams, S. (1998) *Emotions in Social Life: Critical Themes and Contemporary Issues* (London: Routledge).

Benedek, T. (1973) 'Parenthood as a Developmental Phase', in *Psychoanalytic Investigations*, ed. T. Benedek (New York: Quadrangle).

Berger Gluck, S. and Patai, D. (1991) *Women's Words: The Feminist Practice of Oral History* (New York and London: Routledge).

Berger, P. L. and Luckman, T. (1967) *The Social Construction of Reality: A Treatise in the Sociology of Knowledge* (Harmondsworth: Penguin).

Bernardes, J. (1985) 'Family Ideology: Identification and Exploration', *The Sociological Review*, **33**(2), 275–97.

Bertaux, D. (1981) *Biography and Society: The Life History Approach in the Social Sciences* (London: Sage).

Bewley, T. H., Bland, M., Mechen, D. and Walch, E. (1981) '"New Chronic" Patients', *British Medical Journal*, **283**, 254–60.

Biegel, D. E., Sales, E. and Shulz, R. (1990) *Family Caregiving in Chronic Illness* (Newbury Park, Ca.: Sage).

Bittner, E. (1973) 'Objectivity and Realism in Social Science', in G. Psathas (ed.), *Phenomenological Sociology: Issues and Applications* (New York: John Wiley & Sons).

Blaikie, N. (1993) *Approaches to Social Enquiry* (Cambridge: Polity Press).

Bleicher, J. (1982) *The Hermeneutic Imagination: Outline of Positive Critique of Scientism in Sociology* (London: Routledge & Kegan Paul).

Bogdan, R. and Taylor, S. J. (1975) *Introduction to Qualitative Methods: A Phenomenological Approach to the Social Sciences* (New York: John Wiley & Sons).

Bond, J., Coleman, P. and Peace, S. (1993) *Ageing in Society: An Introduction to Social Gerontology* (London: Sage).

Borneman, J. (1996) 'Until Death do us Part: Marriage/Death in Anthropological Discourse', *American Ethnologist*, **23**(2), 215–38.

Bornat, J., Dimmock, B., Jones, D. and Peace, S. (1999) 'The Impact of Family Change on Older People: the Case of Stepfamilies', in S. McRae (ed.), *Changing Britain: Families and Households in the 1990s* (Oxford: Oxford University Press).

Boscolo, L., Gianfanco, C., Hoffman, L. and Penn, P. (1987) *Milan Systemic Family Therapy: Conversations in Theory and Practice* (New York: Basic Books).

Bott, E. (1968) *Family and Social Network* (London: Tavistock Publications).

Bouquet, M. (1996) 'Family Trees and their Affinities: The Visual Imperative of the Genealogical Diagram', *Journal of the Royal Anthropological Institute*, **2**, 43–66.

Bourdieu, P. (1996) 'On the Family as a Realized Category', *Theory, Culture and Society*, **13**(3), 19–26.

Bowen, M. (1960) 'A Family Concept of Schizophrenia', in *The Aetiology of Schizophrenia*, ed. Don Jackson (New York: Basic Books).

Bowlby, J. (1980) *Loss, Sadness and Depression* (London: Hogarth Press).

Boyle, M. (1990) *Schizophrenia: a Scientific Delusion* (London: Routledge).

Brodoff, A. S. (1988) 'First Person Account: Schizophrenia through a Sister's Eyes – the Burden of Invisible Baggage', *Schizophrenia Bulletin*, **14**(1), 113–16.

Broucek, F. J. (1982) 'Shame and its Relationship to Early Narcissistic Developments', *International Journal of Psychoanalysis*, **63**, 369–78.

Brown, G., Bone, M., Dalison, B. and Wing, J. K. (1966) 'Schizophrenia and Social Care: a Comparative Study of 339 Schizophrenic Patients', *Maudsley Monographs*, **17** (London: Oxford University Press).

Brown, S. and Birtwhistle, J. (1998) 'People with Schizophrenia and their Families', *British Journal of Psychiatry*, **173** 139–44.

Brubaker, R. (1984) *The Limits of Rationality: An Essay on the Social and Moral Thought of Max Weber* (London: George Allen Unwin).

Bulmer, M. (1987) *The Social Basis of Community Care* (London: Unwin Hyman).

Burnett, J. A. (1978) *A Social History of Housing, 1815–1970* (Newton Abbott: David and Charles).

Busfield, J. (1974) 'Family Ideology and Family Pathology', in *Reconstructing Social Psychology*, ed. Nigel Armistead (Harmondsworth: Penguin).

—— (1986) *Managing Madness: Changing Ideas and Practice* (London: Hutchinson).

Carrier, J. and Tomlinson, D. (1996) *Asylum in the Community* (London: Routledge).

Casement, P. (1985) *On Learning from the Patient* (London: Tavistock Publications).

—— (1989) *On Further Learning from the Patient* (London: Tavistock Publications).

Castel, R. (1988) *The Regulation of Madness: The Origins of Incarceration in France*, trans. W. D. Hall (Cambridge: Polity Press).

Caton, C. L. (1981) 'The New Chronic Patient and the System of Community Care', *Hospital and Community Psychiatry*, **32** 475–8.

Chassegeut-Smirgel, J. (1985) *The Ego-Ideal* (London: Free Association Books).

Chesler, P. (1972) *Women and Madness* (New York: Avon).

Christie-Brown, J. R. W., Ebringer, L. and Freedman, L. S. (1977) 'A Survey of a Long-stay Psychiatric Population: Implications for Community Services', *Psychological Medicine*, **7**, 113–26.

Cinnirella, M. and Loewenthal, K. M. (1999) 'Religious and Ethnic Group Influences on Beliefs about Mental Illness: A Qualitative Interview Study', *British Journal of Medical Psychology*, **72**, 505–24.

Clare, A. (1976) *Psychiatry in Dissent: Controversial Issues in Thought and Practice* (London: Tavistock Publications).

Clausen, J. A. (1981) 'Stigma and Mental Disorder: Phenomena and Terminology', *Psychiatry: Journal for the Study of Interpersonal Processes*, **44**, 287–96.

Clausen, J. A. and Yarrow, M. R. (1954) 'Mental Illness and the Family', *Journal of Social Issues*, **11**, 3–65.

Colonna, A. B. and Newman, L. M. (1985) 'The Psychoanalytic Literature on Siblings', *Psychoanalytic Study of the Child*, **38**, 285–309.

Conley, R. and Baker, R. (1990) 'Family Response to Improvement by a Relative with Schizophrenia', *Hospital and Community Psychiatry*, **41**(8), 898–901.

Cook, B. and Cohler, B. (1986) 'Reciprocal Socialization and the Case of Offspring with Cancer and Schizophrenia', in N. Datan, A. Green, and

H. Reese, *Life Span Developmental Psychology: Intergenerational Relations* (New York: Academic Press).

Cook, J. A., Pickett, S. A. and Cohler, B. J. (1997) 'Families of Adults with Severe Mental Illness – the Next Generation of Research: Introduction', *American Journal of Orthopsychiatry*, **67**(2), 172–86.

Cournoyer, D. E. and Johnson, H. C. (1991) 'Measuring Parents' Perceptions of Mental Health Professionals', *Research on Social Work Practice*, **1**(4), 399–415.

Cowen, H. (1999) *Community Care, Ideology and Social Policy* (London: Prentice Hall).

Craib, I. (1989) *Psychoanalysis and Social Theory: The Limits of Sociology* (London: Harvester Wheatsheaff).

—— (1995) 'Some Comments on the Sociology of the Emotions', *Sociology*, **29**(1), 151–8.

Creer, C. (1975) 'Living with Schizophrenia', *Social Work Today*, **6**(1), 2–7.

Davis, D. and Schultz, C. (1997) 'Grief, Parenting, and Schizophrenia', *Social Science and Medicine*, **46**(3), 369–79.

Deakin, N. (1987) *The Politics of Welfare* (London: Methuen).

Dell, P. (1989) 'Violence and the Systemic View: the Problem of Power', *Family Process*, **28**, 1–14.

Descombes, V. (1980) *Modern French Philosophy*, trans. L. Scott-Fox, and J. M. Harding (Cambridge: Cambridge University Press).

DHSS (1981) *Care in the Community* (London: HMSO).

Digby, A. (1985) *Madness, Morality and Medicine: A Study of the York Retreat, 1796–1914* (Cambridge: Cambridge University Press).

Dingwall, R., Eekelaar, J. and Murray, T. (1983) *The Protection of Children: State Intervention and Family Life* (Oxford: Basil Blackwell).

Dixon, L. (1997) 'The Next Generation of Research: Views of a Sibling-Psychiatrist-Researcher', *American Journal of Orthopsychiatry*, **67**(2), 242–8.

Dixon, L. and Lehman, A. (1995) 'Family Interventions for Schizophrenia', *Schizophrenia Bulletin*, **21**(4), 631–41.

Doerner, K. (1981) *Madmen and the Bourgeoisie: A Social History of Insanity and Psychiatry* (Oxford: Basil Blackwell).

DoH (1990) *Caring for People: Community Care in the Next Decade and Beyond* (London: HMSO).

—— (1993) *Legal Powers on the Care of Mentally Ill People in the Community: Report of the Internal Review* (London: DoH).

—— (1994) *Introduction of Supervision Registers for Mentally Ill People* (London: DoH).

—— (1995a) *Building Bridges: A Guide to Arrangements for Inter-Agency Working for the Care and Protection of Severely Mentally Ill People* (London: DoH).

—— (1995b) *Carers (Recognition and Services) Act* (London: HMSO).

—— (1995c) *Mental Health (Patients in the Community) Act* (London: HMSO).

Donnolly, M. (1983) *Managing the Mind: A Study of Medical Psychology in Early Nineteenth-Century Britain* (London: Tavistock Publications).

Donzelot, J. (1979) *The Policing of Families* (London: Hutchinson).

Duncombe, J. and Marsden. D. (1993) 'Love and Intimacy: the Gender Division of Emotion and Emotion Work: A Neglected Apect of Sociological Discussion of Heterosexual Relationships', *Sociology*, **27**(2), 221–41.

Eastman, N. (1997) 'The Mental Health (Patients in the Community) Act 1995: A Clinical Analysis', *British Journal of Psychiatry*, **170**, 492–6.

Ebringer, L. and Christie-Brown, J. R. W. (1980) 'Social Deprivation amongst Short Stay Psychiatric Patients', *British Journal of Psychiatry*, **136**, 46–52.

Erikson, E. (1963) *Childhood and Society* (New York: Norton).

—— (1968) *Identity, Youth and Crisis* (New York: Norton).

—— (1982) *The Life-Cycle Completed: A Review* (New York: Norton).

Falloon, I. and Fadden, G. (1993) *Integrated Mental Health Care* (Cambridge: Cambridge University Press).

Fernando, S. (1991) *Mental Health, Race and Culture* (Basingstoke: Macmillan – now Palgrave).

Field, D. (1976) 'The Social Definition of Illness', in *An Introduction to Medical Sociology*, ed. D. Tuckett (London: Tavistock Publications).

Finch, J. (1989) *Family Obligations and Social Change* (Cambridge: Polity Press).

Finch, J. and Groves, D. (1984) 'Community Care and the Family: A Case for Equal Opportunities', *Journal of Social Policy*, **9**, 487–511.

Finch, J. and Mason, J. (1993) *Negotiating Family Responsibilities* (London: Routledge).

Finley, L. Y. (1998) 'The Cultural Context: Families Coping with Severe Mental Illness', *Psychiatric Rehabilitation Journal*, **21**(3), 230–40.

Finnane, M. (1996) 'Law and the Social Uses of the Asylum in Nineteenth-Century Ireland', in J. Carrier and D. Tomlinson (eds), *Asylum in the Community* (London: Routledge).

Fitzpatrick, R. (1989) 'Lay Concepts of Illness', in P. Brown (ed.), *Perspectives in Medical Sociology* (Belmont: Wadsworth Publishing).

Fletcher, J. (1847) 'Moral and Educational Statistics of England and Wales', *Statistical Journal*; cited in H. Perkin (1969), *Origins of Modern English Society* (London: Routledge, and Kegan Paul), p. 161.

Foley, V. (1974) *An Introduction to Family Therapy* (New York: Grune and Stratton).

Foucault, M. (1967) *Madness and Civilisation*, trans. Richard Howard (London: Tavistock Publications).

—— (1974) *The Order of Things: Archaeology of the Human Sciences* (London: Tavistock Publications).

—— (1977) *Discipline and Punish*, trans. Alan Sheridan (New York: Allen Lane).

—— (1979/1990) *The History of Sexuality: Volume 1*, trans. Robert Hurley (Harmondsworth: Penguin).

Fox, L. (1997) 'A Consumer Perspective on the Family Agenda', *American Journal of Orthopsychiatry*, **67**(2), 249–53.

Freeman, H. and Choudrey, M. H. P. (1984) 'Social Characteristics of Newly Admitted Mental Hospital Patients – a Replication Study', *Health Trends*, **16**, 55–7.

Freud, S. (1915) *Introductory Lectures on Psychoanalysis*, Pelican Freud Library, vol. 1 (Harmondsworth: Penguin).

—— (1917) *On Mourning and Melancholia*, in vol. 11, Penguin Freud Library, 'On Metapsychology' (Harmondsworth: Penguin).

—— (1921) *Group Psychology and the Analysis of the Ego*, in vol. 12, Penguin Freud Library, 1991 edn (Harmondsworth: Penguin).

—— (1923) 'The Ego and the Id', in vol. 11, Penguin Freud Library, *On Metapsychology* (Harmondsworth: Penguin).

Fromm-Reichman, F. (1948) 'Notes on Development of Treatment of Schizophrenics by Psychoanalytic Psychotherapy', *Psychiatry*, **11**, 263.

Frosch, S. (1987) *The Politics of Psychoanalysis: An Introduction to Freudian and Post-Freudian Theory* (Basingstoke: Macmillan – now Palgrave).

Furlong, R. (1985) 'Closure of Large Mental Hospitals – Practicable or Desirable', *Bulletin of the Royal College of Psychiatrists*, **9**, 130–4.

Furnham, A. and Bower, P. (1992) 'A Comparison of Academic and Lay Theories of Schizophrenia', *British Journal of Psychiatry*, **161**, 201–10.

Gadamer, H. G. (1975) *Truth and Method* (London: Sheed and Ward).

Gaskell, P. (1836) 'Artisans and Machinery: the Moral and Physical Conditions of the Manufacturing Population', in Perkin (1969), *The Origins of Modern English Society, 1780–1880* (London: Routledge and Kegan Paul).

Giddens, A. (1976) *New Rules of Sociological Method* (London: Basic Books).

—— (1991) *Modernity and Self-Identity* (Cambridge: Polity Press).

—— (1992) *The Transformation of Intimacy* (Cambridge: Polity Press).

Gilbert, P. (1998) 'What is Shame? Some Core Issues and Controversies', in P. Gilbert and B. Andrews (eds), *Shame: Interpersonal Psychopthology and Culture* (Oxford: Oxford University Press).

Gilbert, P. and Andrews, B. (eds) (1998) *Shame: Interpersonal Psychopthology and Culture* (Oxford: Oxford University Press).

Gilbert, P. and McGuire, M. (1998) 'Shame, Status, and Social Roles: Psychobiology and Evolution', in P. Gilbert, and B. Andrews (eds), *Shame: Interpersonal Psychopthology and Culture* (Oxford: Oxford University Press).

Gillis, J. R. (1985) *For Better for Worse: British Marriages, 1600 to the Present* (Oxford: Oxford University Press).

—— (1987) 'From Ritual to Romance: Toward an Alternative History of Love', in *Emotion and Social Change: Towards a New Psychohistory*, ed. C. Stearns and P. Stearns (New York: Holmes and Meir).

Glaser, B. G. and Strauss, A. (1967) *On the Discovery of Grounded Theory* (London: Weidenfeld and Nicolson).

Glennerster, H. and Korman, N. (1985) *Closing a Hospital* (Aldershot: Avebury).

Goetting, A. (1986) 'The Developmental Tasks of Siblingship over the Life-Cycle', *Journal of Marriage and the Family*, **48**, 703–14.

Goffman, E. (1961) *Asylums*, Pelican edn (Harmondsworth: Penguin).

—— (1963) *Stigma: Notes on the Management of Spoiled Identity*, Pelican edn (Harmondsworth: Penguin).

Goldenberg, I. and Goldenberg, H. (1991) *Family Therapy: An Overview* (New York: Academic Press).

Goldie, N. (1986) *'I hated it there but I miss the people': A Study of What has Happened to a Group Ex-long-stay Patients from Claybury Hospital* (London: Health and Social Services Research Unit, South Bank Polytechnic).

Gough, I. (1979) *The Political Economy of the Welfare State* (Basingstoke: Macmillan – now Palgrave).

Grad, J. and Sainsbury, P. (1963) 'Mental Illness and the Family', *The Lancet*, **1**, 544–7.

Greenberg, J. S., Greenley, J. R. and Brown, R. (1997) 'Do Mental Health Services Reduce Stress in Families of People with Serious Mental Illness?', *Psychiatric Rehabilitation Journal*, **21**(1), 40–50.

Greenberg, J. S., Kim, H. W. and Greenley, J. R. (1997) 'Factors Associated with Subjective Burden in Siblings of Adults with Severe Mental Illness', *American Journal of Orthopsychiatry*, **67**(2), 231–41.

Greene, A. L. and Boxer, A. (1986) 'Daughters Issues as Young Adults: Restructuring the Ties that Bind', in N. Datan, A. Green, and H. Reese, *Life Span Developmental Psychology: Intergenerational Relations* (New York: Academic Press).

Griffiths, R. (1988) *Community Care: An Agenda for Action* (London: HMSO).

Grob, G. (1983) *Mental Illness and American Society, 1875–1940* (New Jersey: Princeton University Press).

Gubrium, J. and Holstein, J. (1987) 'The Private Image: Experiential Location and Method in Family Studies', *Journal of Marriage and the Family*, **49**, 773–786.

Guttman, D. (1987) *Reclaimed Powers: Toward a New Psychology of Men and Women in Later Life* (New York: Basic Books).

Hall, P. and Brockington, I. (1991) *The Closure of Mental Hospitals* (London: The Royal College of Psychiatrists).

Harding, C., Brooks, G., Ashikaga, T., Strauss, J. and Brier, A. (1987) 'The Vermont Longitudinal Study of Persons with Severe Mental Illness – parts I and II', *American Journal of Psychiatry*, **144**(6), 718–35.

Harre, R. (1981) 'The Positivist–Empiricist Approach and its Alternative', in J. Rowan and P. Reason (eds), *Human Enquiry: A Source Book for New Paradigm Research* (Chichester: Wiley).

—— (1986) *Varieties of Realism: A Rationale for the Natural Sciences* (Oxford: Blackwell).

Hatfield, A. (1984) 'The Family', in *The Chronic Mental Patient: Five Years Later*, ed. J. Talbot (Orlando, FL: Grune and Stratton).

—— (1987a) 'The Expressed Emotion Theory: Why Families Object', *Hospital and Community Psychiatry*, **38**, 341.

—— (1987b) 'Coping and Adaptation: a Conceptual Framework for Understanding Families', in *Families of the Mentally Ill: Coping and Adaptation*, ed. A. Hatfield, and H. P. Lefley (London: Cassell).

Hatfield, A. and Lefley, H. P. (1987) *Families of the Mentally Ill: Coping and Adaptation* (London: Cassell).

Hatfield, A., Spaniol, L. and Zipple, A. (1987) 'Expressed Emotion: a Family Perspective', *Schizophrenia Bulletin*, **13**(2), 221–5.

Heller, A. (1985) *The Power of Shame* (London: Routledge and Kegan Paul).

Heller, T., Roccoforte, J., Hsieh, K., Cook, J. and Pickett, S. (1997) 'Benefits of Support Groups for Families of Adults with Severe Mental Illness', *American Journal of Orthopsychiatry*, **67**(2), 187–98.

Hill, M. (1993) *The Welfare State in Britain: A Political History since 1945* (Aldershot: Edward Elgar).

Hinshelwood, R. D. (1991) *A Dictionary of Kleinian Thought*, 2nd edn (London: Free Association Books).

Hirsch, S. and Leff, J. (1975) *Abnormalities in the Parents of Schizophrenics* (London: Oxford University Press).

Hirst, D. and Michael, P. (1999) 'Family, Community and the Lunatic in Mid-nineteenth Century North Wales', in P. Bartlett and D. Wright, *Outside the Walls of the Asylum* (London: Athlone Press).

HMSO (1999) *Caring about Carers: A National Strategy for Carers* (London: HMSO).

Hoffman, L. (1981) *Foundations of Family Therapy* (New York: Basic Books).

Holcomb, W. R. and Ahr, P. R. (1987) 'Who Really Treats the Severely Impaired Young Adult Patient? A Comparison of Treatment Settings', *Hospital and Community Psychiatry*, **38**, 625–31.

Holden, D. and Lewine, R. (1982) 'How Families Evaluate Mental Health Professionals, Resources, and Effects of Illness', *Schizophrenia Bulletin*, **8**(4), 626–33.

Hollway, W. (1989) *Subjectivity and Method in Psychology: Gender, Meaning and Science* (London: Sage).

Horwitz, A. (1993) 'Adult Siblings as Sources of Social Support for the Seriously Mentally Ill: A Test of a Serial Model', *Journal of Marriage and the Family* (August) 623–32.

Horwitz, A., Tessler, R., Fisher, G. and Gamache, G. (1992) 'The Role of Adult Siblings in Providing Support to the Seriously Mentally Ill', *Journal of Marriage and the Family*, **54**, 233–41.

Howe, D. (1989) *The Consumer's View of Family Therapy* (Aldershot: Gower).

Hunt, J. (1989) *Psychoanalytic Aspects of Fieldwork*, Qualitative Research Methods, vol. 18 (London: Sage).

Hunter, R. and Macalpine, I. (1963) *Three Hundred Years of Psychiatry, 1535–1860* (Hartdale, NY: Carlisle Publishing).

Illich, I. (1977) *Medical Nemesis: The Expropriation of Health* (New York: Bantam Books).

Ingleby, D. (1985) 'Mental Health and Social Order', in *Social Control and the State*, ed. S. Cohen, and A. Scull (Oxford: Blackwell).

Jacques, E. (1965) 'Death and the Mid-Life Crisis', *International Journal of Psychoanalysis*, **44**, 507–14.

Jenkins, E. (1874) *Glances at Inner England: A Lecture Delivered in the United States and Canada* (London: Henry King).

Jenkins, J. H. and Schumacher, J. G. (1999) 'Family Burden of Schizophrenia and Depressive Illness', *British Journal of Psychiatry*, **174**, 31–8.

Jimenez, M. (1987) *Changing Face of Madness: Early American Attitudes to Treatment of the Insane* (Hanover: University Press of New Hanover).

Jodelet, D. (1991) *Madness and Social Representations*, trans. Tim Pownall (New York: Harvester Wheatsheaf).

Johnson, J. (1975) *Doing Field Research* (New York: The Free Press).

Johnson, M. (1995) 'Interdependency and the Generational Compact', *Ageing and Society*, **15**, 243–65.

Jones, D. (1993) 'The Selection of Patients for Reprovision', *British Journal of Psychiatry*, **162** (supl. 19), 36–9.

Jones, K. (1972) *A History of the Mental Health Services*, 2nd edn (London: Routledge and Kegan Paul).

—— (1982) 'Scull's Dilemma', *British Journal of Psychiatry*, **141**, 221–6.

Kastrup, M. (1987) 'Prediction and Profile of the Long-stay Population', *Acta Psychiatrica Scandinavia*, **76**, 71–9.

Kazarian, S. and Vanderheyden, D. (1992) 'Family Education of Relatives of People with Psychiatric Disability: A Review', *Psychosocial Rehabilitation Journal*, **15**(3), 67–83.

King, M., Coker, E., Leavey, G., Hoare, A. and Johnson-Sabine, E. (1994) 'The Incidence of Psychotic Illness in London: Comparison of Ethnic Groups', *British Medical Journal*, **309**, 1115–9.

King, P. (1974) 'Notes on the Psychoanalysis of Older Patients: Reappraisal of the Potentialities for Change during the Second Half of Life', *Journal of Analytic Psychology*, **19**, 22–37.

—— (1980) 'The Life Cycle as Indicated by the Nature of Transference in the Psychoanalysis of the Middle-aged and Elderly', *International Journal of Psychoanalysis*, **61**, 153–60.

Kingston, W. (1983) 'A Theoretical Context for Shame', *International Journal of Psychoanalysis*, **64**, 213–26.

Kinsella, K. B., Anderson, R. A. and Anderson, W. T. (1996) 'Coping Skills, Strengths, and Needs as Perceived by Adult Offspring of People with Mental Illness: A Retrospective Study', *Psychiatric Rehabilitation Journal*, **20**(2), 24–32.

Klauber, J. (1981) 'The Dual Role of Historical and Scientific Method in Psychoanalysis', reprinted in *Difficulties in the Analytic Encounter*, ed. J. Klauber; originally printed in *International Journal of Psychoanalysis*, (1968) **49**, 80–9.

Klein, M. (1946) 'Notes on Some Schizoid Mechanisms', in *The Selected Melanie Klein*, ed. Juliet Mitchell (Harmondsworth: Penguin, 1986).

Kleinman, S. and Copp, M. A. (1993) *Emotions and Fieldwork*, Qualitative Research Methods, vol. 28 (Newbury Park, Ca: Sage).

Kreisman, D. and Joy, V. (1974) 'Family Response to the Mental Illness of a Relative: a Review of the Literature', *Schizophrenia*, **10**, 34–57.

Kubler-Ross, E. (1973) *On Death and Dying* (London: Tavistock Publications).

Laing, R. D. (1965) *The Divided Self* (Harmondsworth: Penguin).

—— (1967) *The Politics of Experience* (Harmondsworth: Penguin).

Laing, R. D. and Esterson, A. (1964) *Sanity, Madness and the Family* (London: Tavistock).

Lamb, H. and Sutton-Smith, B. (1982) *Sibling Relationships: Their Nature and Significance Across the Life-span* (Hillsdale: Lawrence Erlbaum).

Lambert, H. and Sevak, L. (1996) 'Is Cultural Difference a Useful Concept? Perceptions of Health and the Sources of Ill Health Amongst Londoners of South Asian Origin', in *Researching Cultural Differences in Health*, ed. D. Kelleher and S. Hillier (London: Routledge).

The Lancet (1982) 'Psychiatric Patients who Stick', editorial, 20 November.

Land, H. (1978) 'Who Cares for the Family?', *Journal of Social Policy*, **7**, 257–84.

Lanquetot, R. (1988) 'First Person Account: On Being Daughter and Mother', *Schizophrenia Bulletin*, **14**(2), 335–41.

Laplanche, J. and Pontalis, J. B. (1988) *The Language of Psychoanalysis* (London: Karnac).

Laslett, P. and Wall, R. (1972) *Household and Family in Past-times* (Cambridge: Cambridge University Press).

Lawson, M. (1991) 'A Recipient's View', in S. Ramon (ed.), *Beyond Community Care: Normalisation and Integration Work* (Basingstoke: Macmillan – now Palgrave).

Lee, T. R., Mancini, J. A. and Maxwell, J. W. (1990) 'Sibling Relationships in Adulthood: Contact Patterns and Motivations', *Journal of Marriage and the Family*, **52**, 431–40.

Leff, J. (1994) 'Working with Families of Schizophrenic Patients', *British Journal of Psychiatry*, **164** (suppl 23), 71–6.

Leff, J. and Vaughan, C. (1985) *Expressed Emotion* (London: Guilford).

Lefley, H. (1997) 'The Consumer Recovery Vision: Will it Alleviate Family Burden?', *American Journal of Orthopsychiatry*, **67**(2), 210–19.

Levinson, D., Darrow, C., Klein, E., Levinson, M. and McKee, B. (1978) *The Seasons of a Man's Life* (New York: Ballantine).

Lévi-Strauss, C. (1968) *Structural Anthropology*, trans. Claire Jacobson and Brooke Grundfest Schoepf (Harmondsworth: Penguin).

—— (1969) *The Elementary Structures of Kinship*, trans. J. Harle Beell, J. R. von Strumer, and R. Needham (Boston, MA: Beacon Press).

Lewis, J. (1984) *Women in England, 1870–1950: Sexual Divisions and Social Change* (Hemel Hempstead: Harvester Wheatsheaff).

—— (1992) *Women in Britain since 1945* (Oxford: Blackwell).

Lewis, J. and Meredith, B. (1988) *Daughters Who Care: Daughters Caring for Mothers at Home* (London: Routledge).

Lewis, M. (1998) 'Shame and Stigma', in *Shame: Interpersonal Behaviour, Psychopathology, and Culture*, ed. P. Gilbert, and B. Andrews (Oxford: Oxford University Press).

Lidz, T. (1963) *The Family and Human Adaptation* (New York: International University Press).

Lidz, R. and Lidz, T. (1949) 'The Family Environment of the Schizophrenic Patient', *American Journal of Psychiatry*, **106**, 332–45.

Littlewood, J. (1992) *Aspects of Grief: Bereavement in Adult Life* (London: Tavistock/Routledge).

Littlewood, R. and Lipsedge, M. (1989) *Aliens and Alienists: Ethnic Minorities and Psychiatry*, 2nd edn (London: Unwin Hyman).

Lloyd, L. (2000) 'Caring about Carers: Only Half the Picture?', *Critical Social Policy*, **20**(1), 136–50.

Lowenfeld, H. (1976) 'Notes on Shamelessness', *Psychiatric Quarterly*, **45**, 62–72.

Luhman, N. (1986) *Love as Passion* (Cambridge: Polity Press).

McCreadie, R. G., Wilson, A. O. A. and Burton, L. L. (1983) 'The Scottish Survey of "New Chronic" Inpatients', *British Journal of Psychiatry*, **143**, 564–71.

MacCarthy, B., Lesage, A., Brewin, C. R., Brugha, T., Mangen, S. and Wing, J. (1989) 'Needs for Care amongst the Relatives of Long-term Users of Day Care', *Psychological Medicine*, **19**, 725–36.

McCourt-Perring, C. (1993) *The Experience of Hospital Closure* (Aldershot: Avebury).

MacDonald, J. (1998) 'Disclosing Shame', in P. Gilbert, and B. Andrews, *Shame: Interpersonal Psychopthology and Culture* (Oxford: Oxford University Press).

MacDonald, M. (1981) *Mystical Bedlam: Madness, Anxiety and Healing in Seventeenth-Century England* (Cambridge: Cambridge University Press).

Macfarlane, A. (1986) *Marriage and Love in England: Modes of Reproduction, 1380–1840* (Oxford: Basil Blackwell).

MacGregor, P. (1994) 'Grief: The Unrecognised Parental Response to Mental Illness in a Child', *Social Work* (USA), **39**(2), 161–6.

McKenna, P. J. (1997) *Schizophrenia and Related Syndromes* (Hove: Psychology Press).

MacKenzie, C. (1992) *Psychiatry for the Rich: A History of Ticehurst Private Asylum, 1792–1917* (London: Routledge).

McRae, S. (1999) *Changing Britain: Families and Households in the 1990s* (Oxford: Oxford University Press).

Malan, D. (1979) *Individual Psychotherapy and the Science of Psychodynamics* (London: Butterworth).

Mallon, J. (2000) 'Home, Schizophrenic, Home', unpublished BSc dissertation, Buckinghamshire Chilterns University College.

Malpass, P. and Murie, A. (1987) *Housing Policy and Practice* (London: Macmillan – now Palgrave).

Mann, S. A. and Cree, W. (1976) 'New Long-Stay Psychiatric Patients: a National Sample Survey of Fifteen Mental Hospitals in England and Wales, 1972/3', *Psychological Medicine*, **6**, 603–16.

Mannion, E., Meisel, M., Solomon, P. and Draine, J. (1996) 'A Comparative Analysis of Families with Mentally Ill Adult Relatives: Support Group Members Versus Non-Members', *Psychiatric Rehabilitation Journal*, **20**(1), 43–50.

Marris, P. (1978) *Loss and Change* (London: Routledge and Kegan Paul).

Mashal, M., Feldman, R. and Sigal, J. (1989) 'The Unravelling of a Treatment Paradigm: A Follow-up Study of the Milan Approach to Family Therapy', *Family Process*, **28**, 457–70.

Mason, J. (1994) 'Gender, Care and Sensibility in Family and Kin Relationships', paper presented to the British Sociological Association Annual Conference, *Sexualities in Context*, University of Central Lancashire, Preston, UK, 28–31 March 1994.

Mathieson, C. M. (1999) 'Interviewing the Ill and the Healthy: Paradigm or Process', in *Qualitative Health Psychology: Theories and Methods*, ed. M. Murray and K. Chamberlain (London: Sage).

Measey, L. G. and Smith, H. (1973) 'Patterns of New Chronicity in a Mental Hospital', *British Journal of Psychiatry*, **123**, 349–51.

Menzies Leith, I. (1988) *Containing Anxieties in Institutions* (London: Free Association Books).

Merrell Lynd, H. (1958) *On Shame and the Search for Identity* (New York: Harvester).

Midwinter, E. (1994) *The Development of Social Welfare in Britain* (Buckingham: Open University Press).

Miller, P. (1986) 'Critiques of Psychiatry and Critical Sociologies of Madness', in P. Miller, and N. Rose, *The Power of Psychiatry* (Cambridge: Polity Press).

Mills, E. (1962) *Living with Mental Illness: A Study in East London* (London: Routledge and Kegan Paul).

Mishler, E. (1981) 'The Social Construction of Illness', in *Social Contexts of Health, Illness, and Patient Care*, ed. E. G. Mishler, L. Amarasingham, S. D. Osherson, S. T. Hauser, N. E. Waxler and R. Liem (Cambridge: Cambridge University Press).

Moorman, M. (1992) 'My Sister's Keeper' (New York: Norton). Quoted in E. F. Torrey (ed.), *Surviving Schizophrenia: A Manual for Families, Consumers and Providers* (1995) (New York: Harper Perennial).

Mosher, L. and Burti, R. (1989) *Community Mental Health: Principles and Practice* (New York: Norton).

Muijen, M. (1996) 'Scare in the Community: Britain in Moral Panic', in *Mental Health Matters*, ed. T. Heller, J. Reynolds, R. Gomm, R. Muston, and S. Pattison (Basingstoke: Macmillan – now Palgrave).

Murphy, E. (1991) *After the Asylums: Community Care for People with Mental Illness* (London: Faber).

Murray Parkes, C. (1972) *Bereavement: Studies of Grief in Adult Life* (London: Tavistock).

Nathason, D. (1987) *The Many Faces of Shame* (London and New York: The Guilford Press).

Nicholls, M. P. and Schwartz, R. C. (1991) *Family Therapy: Concepts and Methods* (Boston: Allyn and Bacon).

Oakley, A. (1981) 'Interviewing Women: A Contradiction in Terms', in *Doing Feminist Research*, ed. H. Roberts (London: Routledge and Kegan Paul).

O'Connell Davidson, J. and Laydor, D. (1994) *Methods, Sex and Madness* (London: Routledge and Kegan Paul).

Parkin, A. (1996) 'Caring for Patients in the Community: Mental Health (Patients in the Community) Act 1995', *Modern Law Review*, **59**, 414–26.

Parsons, T. (1955) 'The American Family: Its Relations to Personality and to the Social Structure', in T. Parsons and R. Bales (eds), *Family, Socialization and Interaction Process* (New York: The Free Press).

Parsons, T. and Bales, R. (1955) *Family, Socialization and Interaction Process* (New York: The Free Press).

Parton, N. (1991) *Governing the Family: Child Care, Child Protection and the State* (Basingstoke: Macmillan – now Palgrave).

Pepper, B., Kirshner, M. C. and Ryglewicz, H. (1981) 'The Young Adult Chronic Patient: Overview of a Population', *Hospital and Community Psychiatry*, **32**, 463–69.

Pepper, B., Ryglewicz, H. and Kirshner, M. C. (1982) 'The Uninstitutionalised Generation: A New Breed of Psychiatric Patient', in *The Young Adult Chronic Patient: New Directions for Mental Health Services*, **14**, ed. B. Pepper and H. Ryglewicz (San Francisco: Jossey Bass).

Perelberg, R. (1983a) 'Family and Mental Illness in a London Borough', PhD. thesis, University of London.

—— (1983b) 'Mental Illness, Family and Networks in a London Borough: Two Cases Studied by an Anthropologist', *Social Science and Medicine*, **17**(8), 481–91.

Perelberg, R. and Miller, A. L. (1990) *Gender and Power in Families* (London: Routledge).

Perkin, H. (1969) *The Origins of Modern English Society, 1780–1880* (London: Routledge and Kegan Paul).

Perring, C. (1990) 'Leaving the Hospital Behind? An Anthropological Study of Group Homes in Two London Boroughs', PhD thesis, University of London.

—— (1992) 'The Experience of Perspectives of Patients and Care Staff of the Transition from the Hospital to the Community-based Care', in S. Ramon,

Psychiatric Hospital Closure: Myths and Realities (London: Chapman and Hall).

Perring, C., Twigg, J. and Atkin, K. (1990) *Families Caring for People Diagnosed as Mentally Ill: The Literature Re-examined* (London: HMSO).

Phillips, R. (1988) *Putting Asunder: A History of Divorce in Western Society* (Cambridge: Cambridge University Press).

Pick, D. (1989) *Faces of Degeneration: A European Disorder, 1848–1918* (Cambridge: Cambridge University Press).

Pickett, S., Cook, J., Cohler, B. and Solomon, M. (1997) 'Positive Parent/Adult Child Relationships: Impact of Severe Mental Illness and Caregiving Burden', *American Journal of Orthopsychiatry*, **67**(2), 220–30.

Piers, G. and Singer, M. B. (1953) *Shame and Guilt: A Psychoanalytic and Cultural Study* (Springfield, Ill: W. W. North).

Pilgrim, D. and Rogers, A. (1993) *A Sociology of Mental Health* (Buckingham: Open University Press).

Platt, S. (1985) 'Measuring the Burden of Psychiatric Illness on the Family: An Evaluation of Some Rating Scales', *Psychological Medicine*, **15**, 383–93.

Plummer, K. (1995) *Telling Sexual Stories* (London: Routledge).

Poponoe, D. (1988) *Disturbing the Nest: Family Change and Decline in Modern Societies* (New York: Arde Grutyer).

—— (1993) 'American Family Decline, 1960–1990: a Review and Appraisal', *Journal of Marriage and the Family*, **55**, 9527–55.

Porter, R. (1987) *Mind-forg'd Manacles* (Harmondsworth: Penguin).

Poster, M. (1978) *Critical Theory of the Family* (London: Pluto Press).

Potter, J. and Wetherell, M. (1987) *Discourse and Social Psychology: Beyond Attitudes and Behaviour* (London: Sage).

Prior, L. (1996) 'The Appeal to Madness in Ireland', in J. Carrier, and D. Tomlinson (eds), *Asylum in the Community* (London: Routledge).

Ramon, S. (1985) *Psychiatry in Britain: Meaning and Policy* (Kings Lynne: Croom Helm).

—— (1991) *Beyond Community Care: Normalisation and Integration Work* (Basingstoke: Macmillan – now Palgrave).

—— (1992) *Psychiatric Hospital Closure: Myths and Realities* (London: Chapman and Hall).

Raphael-Leff, J. (1991) *Psychological Processes of Child-Bearing* (London: Routledge).

Raynor, E. (1991) *The Independent Mind in Psychoanalysis* (London: Free Association Books).

Reed, J. and Reynolds, J. (1996) *Speaking Our Minds: An Anthology* (Basingstoke: Macmillan – now Palgrave).

Reimers, S. and Treacher, S. (1995) *Introducing User-Friendly Family Therapy* (London: Routledge).

Retzinger, S. (1998) 'Shame in the Therapeutic Relationship', in P. Gilbert and B. Andrews (eds), *Shame: Interpersonal Psychopthology and Culture* (Oxford: Oxford University Press).

Richardson, L. (1990) *Writing Strategies: Reaching Diverse Audiences*, Qualitative Research Methods Series, 21 (Newbury Park, Ca: Sage).

Rizzuto, A.-M. (1991) 'Shame in Psychoanalysis: the Function of Unconscious Fantasies', *International Journal of Psychoanalysis*, **72**, 297–312.

Robb, B. (1967) *Sans Everything: A Case to Answer* (London: Nelson).

Robertson Elliot, F. (1996) *Gender, Family and Society* (Basingstoke: Macmillan – now Palgrave).

Robinson, E. A. R. (1996) 'Causal Attributions about Mental Illness: Relationship to Family Functioning', *American Journal of Orthopsychiatry*, **66**(2), 282–95.

Rogers, M. (1983) *Sociology, Ethnomethodology, and Experience: A Phenomenological Critique* (Cambridge: Cambridge University Press).

Rogers, A., Pilgrim, D. and Lacey, A. (1993) *Experiencing Psychiatry: Users' Views of Services* (London: Macmillan and MIND).

Rorty, R. (1980) *Philosophy and the Mirror of Nature* (Oxford: Basil Blackwell).

—— (1991) *Essays on Heidegger and Others* (Cambridge: Cambridge University Press).

Rose, N. (1986) 'Psychiatry: the Discipline of Mental Health', in P. Miller and N. Rose (eds), *The Power of Psychiatry* (Cambridge: Polity Press).

—— (1989) *Governing the Soul: The Shaping of the Private Self* (London: Routledge).

Rothman, D. J. (1971) *The Discovery of the Asylum* (Toronto: Little, Brown).

Rud, J. and Noreik, K. (1982) 'Who Became Long-stay Patients in a Psychiatric Hospital', *Acta Scandinavia*, **65**, 1–14.

Rycroft, C. (1968) 'An Enquiry into the Function of Words', in G. Kohon, *The British School of Psychoanalysis: The Independent Tradition* (London: Faber).

Sandler, J., Dare, C. and Holder, A. (1973) *The Patient and the Analyst: The Basis of the Psychoanalytic Process* (London: Karnac).

Scheff, T. J. (1966) *Being Mentally Ill: A Sociological Theory* (London: Weidenfeld and Nicolson).

—— (1975) *Labelling Madness* (Englewood Cliff, NJ: Prentice Hall).

—— (1990) *Microsociology: Discourse, Emotion, and Social Structure* (London: University of Chicago Press).

—— (1998) 'Shame in the Labelling of Mental Illness', in *Shame: Interpersonal Behaviour, Psychopathology, and Culture*, ed. P. Gilbert, and B. Andrews (Oxford: Oxford University Press).

Schneider, D. (1980) *American Kinship: A Cultural Account*, 2nd edn (Chicago and London: University of Chicago Press).

—— (1984) *A Critique of the Study of Kinship* (Ann Arbor: University of Michigan Press).

Schutz, A. (1954) 'Concept and Theory Formation in the Social Sciences', repr. in K. Thompson and J. Tunstall, *Sociological Perspectives* (Harmondsworth: Penguin).

—— (1967) *The Phenomenology of the Social World*, trans. G. Walsh and F. Lehnert (Evanston, Ill.: North Western University Press).

Schwartz, S. R. and Goldfinger, S. M. (1981) 'The New Chronic Patient: Clinical Characteristics of an Emerging Sub-group', *Hospital and Community Psychiatry*, **32**, 470–4.

Scott, R. D. (1973) 'The Treatment Barrier: Part 2. The Patient as an Unrecognised Agent', *British Journal of Medical Psychology*, **46**, 57–67.

Scott, R. D. and Ashworth, P. L. (1967) 'Closure at the First Schizophrenic Break-down: a Family Study', *British Journal of Medical Psychology*, **40**, 109–45.

The Scottish Schizophrenia Research Group (1987) 'The Scottish First Episode Schizophrenia Study: IV. Psychiatric and Social Impact on Relatives', *British Journal of Psychiatry*, **150**, 340–4.

Scull, A. (1979) *Museums of Madness* (London: Allen Lane).

—— (1984) *Decarceration*, 2nd edn (Cambridge: Polity Press).

—— (1989) *Social Disorder/Mental Disorder: Anglo-American Psychiatry in Historical Perspective* (London: Routledge).

Scully, D. (1990) *Understanding Sexual Violence* (London: Harper Collins).

Seccombe, W. (1992) *A Millennium of Family Change: Feudalism to Capitalism in Northwestern Europe* (London: Verso).

Secunda, V (1997) *When Madness Comes Home: Help and Hope for the Families of the Mentally Ill* (New York: Hyperion).

Sedgwick, P. (1982) *Psycho Politics* (London: Pluto Press).

Segal, H. (1952) 'A Psychoanalytical Approach to Aesthetics', *International Journal of Psychoanalysis*, **33**, 196–207.

Segal, J. (1991) 'The Professional Perspective', in S. Ramon (ed.), *Beyond Community Care: Normalisation and Integration Work* (Basingstoke: Macmillan – now Palgrave).

Selvini-Palozzoli, M., Boscolo, L., Cecchin, G. and Prati, C. (1978) *Paradox and Counter-paradox: A New Model in the Therapy of the Family in Schizophrenic Transactions* (New York: Jason Aronson).

Shepherd, G., Murray, A. and Muijen, M. (1994) 'Relative Values: the Differing Views of Users, Family Carers and Professionals on Services for People with Schizophrenia in the Community' (London: The Sainsbury Centre for Mental Health).

Sheridan, A. and Moore, L. (1991) 'Running Groups for Parents with Schizophrenic Adolescents: Initial Experiences and Plans for the Future', *Journal of Adolescence*, **14**, 1–16.

Silva, E. and Smart, C. (1999) *The New Family* (London: Sage).

Silverman, D. (1985) *Qualitative Methodology and Sociology* (Brookfield: Gower Publishing).

—— (1993) *Interpreting Qualitative Data: Methods for Analysing Talk, Text, and Interaction* (London: Sage).

Simmons, S. (1990) 'Family Burden – What Does Psychiatric Illness Mean to the Carer?', in *Community Psychiatric Nursing: A Research Perspective*, ed. C. Brooker (London: Chapman and Hall).

Skultans, V. (1975) *Madness and Morals: Ideas on Insanity in the Nineteenth Century* (London: Routledge).

—— (1979) *English Madness: Ideas on Insanity, 1580–1890* (London: Routledge).

Smith, J. A., Jarman, M. and Osborn, M. (1999) 'Doing Interpretive Phenomenological Analysis', in *Qualitative Health Psychology: Theories and Methods*, ed. M. Murray, and K. Chamberlain (London: Sage).

Solomon, P., Driane, J., Mannion, E. and Meisel, M. (1997) 'Effectiveness of Two Models of Brief Family Education: Retention of Gains by Family Members of Adults with Serious Mental Illness', *American Journal of Orthopsychiatry*, **67**(2), 177–86.

Spaniol, L., Zipple, A. M. and Lockwood, D. (1992) 'The Role of the Family in Psychiatric Rehabilitation', *Schizophrenia Bulletin*, **18**(3), 341–47.

Steiner, J. (1992) 'The Equilibrium Between the Paranoid-Schizoid and the Depressive Position', in *Clinical Lectures on Klein and Bion*, ed. R. Anderson (London: Tavistock/Routledge).

Stearns, C. and Stearns, P. (1988) *Emotion and Social Change: Toward a New Psychohistory* (New York: Holmes and Meier).

Stenson, K. (1993) 'Social Work Discourse and the Social Work Interview', *Economy and Society*, **22**(1), 42–76.

Stone, L. (1977) *The Family, Sex and Marriage in England, 1500–1800* (London: Weidenfeld and Nicolson).

Strathern, M. (1992) *After Nature: English Kinship in the Late Twentieth Century* (Cambridge: Cambridge University Press).

Strauss, A. (1987) *Qualitative Analysis for the Social Sciences* (Cambridge: Cambridge University Press).

Strong, S. (1997) *Unconditional Love: The Views and Experiences of Parents Living with Children with Mental Health Problems* (London: The Mental Health Foundation).

Stueve, A., Vine, P. and Strueng, E. L. (1997) 'Perceived Burden among Caregivers of Adults with Serious Mental Illness: Comparison of Black, Hispanic and White Families', *American Journal of Orthopsychiatry*, **67**(2), 199–209.

Sullivan, P. (1998) 'Progress or Neglect? Reviewing the Impact of Care in the Community for the Severely Mentally Ill', *Critical Social Policy*, **18**(2), 193–213.

Suzuki, A. (1999) 'Enclosing and Disclosing Lunatics within the Family Walls: Domestic Psychiatric Regime and the Public Sphere in Early 19th Century England', in P. Bartlett and D. Wright, *Outside the Asylum Walls* (London: Athlone Press).

Szasz, T. (1970) *The Manufacture of Madness* (New York: Harper and Row).

TAPS (1989) *Moving Long-Stay Psychiatric Patients into the Community: First Results* (London: NETRHA).

—— (1990) *Better Out than In?*, Report of 5th Annual TAPS Conference (London: NETRHA).

Tarrier, N. (1996) 'Family Interventions in Schizophrenia', in G. Haddock, and P. Slade (eds), *Cognitive–Behavioural Intervention with Psychotic Disorders* (London: Routledge).

Taylor, C. (1989) *Sources of the Self: The Making of Modern Identity* (Cambridge: Cambridge University Press).

Terkelsen, K. G. (1987) 'The Meaning of Mental Illness to the Family', in *Families of the Mentally Ill: Coping and Adaptation*, ed. A. Hatfield, and H. Lefley (London: Cassell).

Thornicroft, G., Margolius, O. and Jones, D. (1993) 'New Long-stay Psychiatric Patients and Social Deprivation', *British Journal of Psychiatry*, **161**, 621–4.

Thrane, G. (1979) 'Shame and the Construction of the Self', *The Annual of Psychoanalysis*, **vii**, 321–41.

Timms, N. (1964) *Psychiatric Social Work in Great Britain (1939–1962)* (London: Routledge and Kegan Paul).

Todd, N. A., Bennie, E. H., and Carlisle, J. M., (1976) 'Some Features of "New Long-stay" Male Schizophrenics', *British Journal of Psychiatry*, **129**, 424–7.

Tomes, N. (1994) *The Art of Asylum-Keeping: Thomas Story Kirkbride and the Origins of American Psychiatry* (Pennsylvania: University of Pennsylvania Press).

Tomlinson, D. (1992) *Utopia, Community Care and the Retreat from the Asylums* (Buckingham: Open University Press).

Tooth, G. C. and Brooke, E. M. (1961) 'Trends in the Mental Hospital Population and Their Effect on Future Planning', *Lancet*, 1 April, 710–13.

Tsuang, M. T. and Vandermey, R. (1980) *Genes and the Mind: Inheritance of Mental Illness* (Oxford: Oxford University Press).

Turner, B. and Rennell, T. (1995) *When Daddy Came Home: How Family Life Changed Forever in 1945* (London: Pimlico).

Ungerson, C. (1990) *Gender and Caring: Work and Welfare in Britain and Scandinavia* (London: Harvester Wheatsheaff).

Vaillant, G. (1977) *Adaptation to Life* (Boston, MA: Little, Brown).

Vaughan, P. J. (1998) 'Supervision Register in Practice', *Psychiatric Bulletin*, **22**, 412–15.

Vogler, C. (2000) 'Social Identity and Emotion: the Meeting of Psychoanalysis and Sociology', *The Sociological Review*, **48**, 19–42.

Wahl, O. F. and Harman, C. R. (1989) 'Family Views of Stigma', *Schizophrenia Bulletin*, **15**(1), 131–9.

Walton J. K. (1985) 'Casting Out and Bringing Back in Victorian England: Pauper Lunatics, 1840–70', in *The Anatomy of Madness*, ed. T. Bynum, R. Porter, and M. Shepherd (London and New York: Tavistock).

Warner, R. (1985) *Recovery from Schizophrenia* (London: Routledge).

Wasow, M. (1995) *The Skipping Stone: Ripple Effects of Mental Illness on the Family* (Palo Alto, Ca.: Science and Behaviour Books).

Weeks, J. (1981) *Sex, Politics and Society* (London: Longman).

Weeks, J., Heaphy, B. and Donovan, C. (1999) 'Families of Choice: Autonomy and Mutuality in Non-heterosexual Relationships', in S. McRae, *Changing Britain: Families and Households in the 1990s* (Oxford: Oxford University Press).

Weller, M. (1985) 'Psychiatric Hospital Closures', Correspondence, *Bulletin of British Psychological Society*, December 1985.

Wertheimer, A. (1991) *A Special Scar: The Experiences of People Bereaved by Suicide* (London: Routledge).

Williams, G. and Popay, J. (1994) 'Lay Knowledge and the Privilege of Experience', in *Challenging Medicine*, ed. J. Gabe, D. Kelleher, and G. Williams, (London: Routledge).

Willick, M. S. (1994) 'Schizophrenia: a Parent's Perspective – Mourning without End', in *Schizophrenia: From Mind to Molecule*, ed. N. C. Andreasen and A. H. Woods (Washington: American Psychiatric Press).

Willis, M. J. (1982) 'The Impact of Schizophrenia on Families: One Mother's Point of View', *Schizophrenia Bulletin*, **8**(4), 617–19.

Wilson, E. (1977) *Women and the Welfare State* (London: Tavistock Publications).

Winefield, H. R. and Harvey, E. J. (1994) 'Needs of Family Caregivers in Chronic Schizophrenia', *Schizophrenia Bulletin*, **20**(3), 557–66.

Wolfram, S. (1987) *In-Laws and Outlaws: Kinship and Marriage in England* (London: Croom Helm).

Wong, D. F. K. (2000) 'Stress Factors and Mental Health of Carers with Relatives Suffering from Schizophrenia in Hong Kong: Implications for Culturally Sensitive Practices', *British Journal of Social Work*, **30**, 365–82.

Wouters, C. (1992) 'On Status Competition and Emotion Management: the Study of Emotions as a New Field', *Theory, Culture and Society*, **9**, 229–52.

Wurmser, L. (1981) *The Mask of Shame* (Baltimore, Md., and London: Johns Hopkins University Press).

Wynne, L., Ryckoff, J. and Hirsch, S. (1958) 'Pseudo-mutuality in the Family Relations of Schizophrenics', *Psychiatry*, **21**, 205–20.

Yarrow, M. R., Green Shwartz, C., Murphy, H. S. and Calhoun Deasy, L. (1954) 'The Psychological Meaning of Mental Illness in the Family', *Journal of Social Issues*, **11**, 12–24.

Young, A. (1981) 'When Rational Men Fall Sick: an Inquiry into Some Assumptions Made by Medical Anthropologists', *Culture, Medicine and Psychiatry*, **5**(4), 317–35.

Zirul, D., Lieberman, A. and Rapp, C. (1989) 'Respite Care for the Chronically Mentally Ill: Focus for the 1990s', *Community Mental Health Journal*, **25**(3), 171–84.

Subject Index

Bold type refers to pages where the topic is dealt with in some detail.

Author Index